THE DIETER'S DICTIONARY

By Victoria Zak
and Peter Vash, MD, MPH
With Deborah D. Reilly

PRODUCTIONS
New Jersey

Dedications & Acknowledgments

I'd like to thank God, and others. My family — Leona Zak, Judy Wagner, Kathy Zak and Katy Lembcke for their love. Mike Kenyon, George Blackburn, MD and Cris Carlin, RD for inspiration. Don Axinn for his remarkable heart. Stacey Chase for her treasured friendship. Joe Borsellino for his kindness. Paul LaFramboise for his gift of insight. Vivian Forlander for the mirror. Blondie and Urse for their purrs. And all the researchers who make food science and weight management a thrill.

Victoria Zak

I'd like to dedicate this book to two very special men in my life, William J. Downs, my father and Michael W. Reilly, my husband. They always said yes you can when the world said no you can't. I give them my heart and thank them for theirs.

Deborah D. Reilly

I'd like to dedicate this book to George, Virginia, Barbara and Stephen Vash.

Peter Vash, MD

International Standard Book Number 0-9628101-0-X

This book is not intended as a prescription, but as a guide to help you make healthy choices. Always see your doctor before you start any diet.

The Dieter's Dictionary
P. O. Box 1255
Brigantine, New Jersey 08203
1-800-962-6990

Segments of Exercise, Protein, Fat, and Carbohydrates are adapted from The Fat-to-Muscle Diet by Victoria Zak, Cris Carlin, MS, RD, and Peter Vash, MD, used with permission.

First Printing 1991
Printed in the United States of America

We would like to thank the following
special people for their support.

Patricia Downs

Joni Johnson

Theresa Bergen Carrigan

Neil Evans

The Dieter's Dictionary

Design & Graphics
by
Patricia T. Berggoetz

introduction

We're happy you own a copy of The Dieter's Dictionary and we think you will be too.

This is the first resource of its kind to give you everything you need to know about weight loss, maintenance, food management and fitness in one easy reference. And that's no easy task, since the science of successful weight control includes many sciences working in harmony. They include diet, exercise, behavior modification, nutrition education, food cue control, lifestyle training, physiology, biochemistry, and psychology.

As a health conscious consumer, you face a difficult task in today's marketplace when you're looking for answers to your most pressing diet or health questions. Your problem is one of information overload and niche-specific programs. More than 400 diet books give you conflicting information about weight loss and maintenance. More than 500 exercise books talk about exercising, either in relationship to a diet, or on its own. More than 500 nutrition books talk about nutrition in relationship to a particular diet, or in an isolated program. Where can you look if you want to get the basic science that is the foundation of diet, exercise, health, nutrition and fitness? Now you have that resource in The Dieter's Dictionary.

But The Dieter's Dictionary is more than an answer-finder. It's an educational aid, a health guide, a companion for support, and a self-empowering resource. It gives you the guidelines you need to make healthy, effective choices. It gives you charts and counters for easy comparisons, how to's for immediate use, and it's based on what you CAN DO, not what you CAN'T DO, so we think it will be a real inspiration for positive change.

This book is about science, but it is also about treating yourself right. Whether you are dieting for weight loss, or specific health needs, such as sodium reduction or cholesterol reduction for a healthy heart, The Dieter's Dictionary is the resource you can turn to for practical, helpful information that will get you on the right track.

The simple fact is, knowledge is power. When you have science on your side, you have the knowledge you need to make sound choices and take an active role in your own program for health or wellbeing. When you are armed with information, it makes you less susceptible to faddish programs and imbalanced food plans that can undermine your fitness goals.

The Dieter's Dictionary is keyed for your easy use:

Food Questions	See Food Keys ●
Behavior Questions	See Behavior Keys ▲
Exercise Questions	See Exercise Keys ◆

You can find easy ways to take charge of your own program with many behavior modification and food management skills. These are indicated by arrows

How To's	See ➠

We also included a key to topics that are particularly vital for heart health. These are keyed with a heart.

Heart Health	See ❤

That's all you need to know to get started.

ON A DIET, use it to fill in the gaps in your program.

OFF A DIET, use it to eat healthy.

NEED A DIET, use the scientific one that is the basis of all healthy programs in the country. You'll find it in FOOD GROUPS.

We hope you enjoy The Dieter's Dictionary. It's a resource about you — trusting in yourself and believing in your own unique individuality, and how you can enhance that to feel really good about yourself and your health. It's also about changing the way we diet in America.

Our best to you,
The Authors

a

ABSORPTION, CALORIE The process between digestion and metabolism where nutrients are absorbed by your blood. During digestion, your food nutrients are broken down into smaller and smaller molecules to convert them into the form that your blood can absorb. Carbohydrates are broken down into glucose, Fat into fatty acids and glycerol, protein into amino acids. This process starts in your mouth and ends in your small intestines where absorption takes place. When the nutrients are in the form that your blood can pick up, they pass into the cells of your intestinal lining. From there, they are absorbed into your bloodstream and lymphatic system. Some nutrients go to your liver for storage, to be metered out when you need them. Other nutrients go to your adipose tissue to be stored and metered out when you need them. The rest go to all the cells of your body for the process of metabolism. *See* Digestion. Metabolism.

ACIDITY An acidic system. This is often the result of gastric juices that are not neutralized after digestion. It can be prevented by eating a more fibrous diet, rather than taking a medication. Fiber binds with bile acids and excess bile is excreted. The double benefit for a dieter is better weight loss, since high fiber diets lead to less fat storage. *See* Fiber.

ADDITIVES Chemical, synthetic or natural ingredients added to foods for a variety of purposes, such as coloring, flavoring, sweetening, preserving, emulsifying, thickening and chelating.

Excess additives aren't good for anyone, but particularly not for dieters. When you are on a calorie-limited plan, your system is more susceptible to foreign substances, and you can experience symptoms you might not have otherwise. Real fresh food is the best way to burn fat, protect your body muscle and re-vitalize your health. Foods with additives are typically low-nutrition foods with added fats, sugars, salt, and little or no fiber. That's the combination that leads to weight gain. So you'll find that a non-additive diet is also a fat-prevention technique that's automatic.

To choose the best foods, look for products with natural additives that are safe or even beneficial. For instance, beta carotene, used as a coloring agent is a valuable source of Vitamin A, and lecithin, used as an emulsifier is a good source of choline.

Over-processed foods need additives to try to fix the problems created by processing — loss of color and texture, lack of stabilization, loss of appeal. Often they need additional additives to counterbalance harmful effects inherent in one of the additives they used. For instance, sodium nitrate and nitrite in bacon, ham and cured meats is known to form potent carcinogens called nitrosamines. To prevent nitrosamines from forming, ascorbic acid is needed as an additive. It makes sense chemically, but you don't need to take the risk with your body.

When you start tracking additives on your supermarket shelves, and see the overwhelming number of foods that use long lists of additives, it will give you a new respect for the companies that had your welfare in mind when they opted for natural or safe additives.

ADDITIVES. WHAT TO LOOK FOR ON FOOD LABELS

ANTIOXIDANTS Prevent rancidity, loss of color and flavor.

	CHEMICAL	
Butylated Hydroxytoluene (BHT)	Cereals Gums Chips	Avoid May Promote Cancer, Allergies
Butylated Hydroxyanisole (BHA)	Cereals Gums Chips Oils	Avoid Not Enough Tests
Propyl Gallate	Soup Bases Meat Products Oils	Avoid Not Enough Tests
	NATURAL	
Alpha Tocopherol (Vitamin E)	Wheats Rices Oils	Beneficial
Ascorbic Acid (Vitamin C)	Cereals Meats Sodas Oily Foods	Beneficial
Lecithin	Baked Goods Margarine Chocolate Ice Cream	Beneficial

ADDITIVES. WHAT TO LOOK FOR ON FOOD LABELS

CHELATORS Trap metal atoms that cause food to spoil.

	NATURAL	
Citric Acid	Ice Cream	Safe
	Sherbet	
	Fruit Drinks	
	Candy	
	Instant Potatoes	
EDTA	Salad Dressings	Safe
	Margarines	
	Mayo	
	Processed Fruit	
	Processed Veg	
	Soft Drinks	
	Canned Shellfish	

	NATURAL	
Phosphoric Acid	Baked Goods	Avoid
Phosphates	Cured Meats	Excess Can Lead
	Sodas	To Osteoporosis
	Cereals	
	Cheese	

COLORINGS To make food look palatable.

	CHEMICAL	
Blue #1	Sodas	Not Safe
	Candy	Poorly Tested
	Baked Goods	
Blue #2	Sodas	Not Safe
	Candy	Tumors in Rats

ADDITIVES. WHAT TO LOOK FOR ON FOOD LABELS

Red #2	Some Florida Orange Skins	Not Safe Cancerous
Red #3	Cherries Candy Baked Foods	Not Safe Cancer
Red #40	Sodas Candy Baked Goods Sausage	Questionable
Green #3	Sodas Candy	Not Safe Tumors in Rats
Yellow #5	Candy Baked Goods Gelatins	Not Safe Poorly Tested May Promote Cancer, Allergies
Yellow #6	Sodas Candy Baked Goods Sausage	Appears Safe But Watch Allergies
	NATURAL	
Beta Carotene	Margarine Shortening Creamers Butter	Beneficial
Ferrous Glutonate	Black Olives Pills	Beneficial
Dextrose Glucose	Breads Baked Goods	Safe Empty Calories

ADDITIVES. WHAT TO LOOK FOR ON FOOD LABELS

EMULSIFIERS Keeps oils and water from separating.

	CHEMICAL	
Polysorbate 60	Baked Goods Imitation Dairy Frozen Desserts Pickles	Not Pure Can Contain Carcinogenic Compounds
Sorbitan	Desserts Candy Icings	Safe
	NATURAL	
Bromated Vegetable Oil (BVO)	Soft Drinks	Avoid Not Tested Enough
Lecithin	Margarine Baked Goods Ice Cream Chocolate	Beneficial
Monoglycerides Diglycerides	Baked Goods Peanut Butter Candy Margarine	Safe
Phosphoric Acid Phosphates	Cereals Sodas Baked Goods Cheese Processed Foods	Excess Can Lead To Osteoporosis

ADDITIVES. WHAT TO LOOK FOR ON FOOD LABELS

FLAVORINGS Chemicals that imitate natural flavors. Often many chemicals are needed to make one flavor.

CHEMICAL		
More Than 100	Sodas Candy Cereals Gelatins	Can Cause Hyperactivity In Children
Ethyl Vanillin	Ice Cream Baked Goods Chocolate Candy Gelatins	Needs Testing
Quinine	Tonic Waters Bitters	Can Cure Malaria Not For Pregnant Women Poorly Tested
Sodium Nitrate Sodium Nitrite	Cured Meats Lunch Meats Bacon Ham Hot Dogs	Promotes Cancer Causing Nitrosamines
NATURAL		
Citric Acid	Ice Cream Sherbet Fruit Drinks Candy Carbonated Drinks Instant Potatoes	Safe

ADDITIVES. WHAT TO LOOK FOR ON FOOD LABELS

Sodium Citrate	Ice Cream Candy Jams	Safe
Fumaric Acid	Powdered Drinks Puddings Pie Fillings Gelatins	Safe Not Great Needs Detergent-like Additive To Dissolve in Cold Water
Ethyl Vanillin	Ice Cream Baked Goods Sodas Chocolate Candy	Safe
Hydrolyzed Vegetable Protein (HUP)	Instant Soups Hot Dogs Sauces Stews	Beneficial
MSG Monosodium Glutomate	Processed Foods Soups Stews Poultry Seafood	Avoid Affects Nerve Cells In Brain MSG Syndrome
Sodium Chloride	Most Processed Foods	Excess Can Cause High Blood Pressure

ADDITIVES. WHAT TO LOOK FOR ON FOOD LABELS

PRESERVATIVES Prevent mold and bacteria.

CHEMICAL		
Sulfur Dioxide	Processed Fruits Instant Potatoes Wine	Safe But Destroys Vitamin B-1
NATURAL		
Calcium Propionate Sodium Propionate	Baked Goods	Safe
Heptyl Paraben	Beer Poorly Tested	Safe
Sodium Benzoate	Fruit Juices Pickles Preserves	Safe But Excess Causes High Blood Pressure
Sodium Nitrate Sodium Nitrite	Bacon Lunch Meats Cured Meats	Not Safe Carcinogenic Nitrosamines Created
Sorbic Acid	Cheese Baked Goods Syrups Dried Fruits Wines	Safe

ADDITIVES. WHAT TO LOOK FOR ON FOOD LABELS

SWEETENERS Add sweet taste.
Brown Sugar, Caramel, Corn Syrup, Corn Syrup Solids, Dextrose, Fructose, Glucose, Honey, Lactate, Maltose, Malitol, Mannitol, Raw Sugar, Sorbitol, Sucrose, Turbinado, Xylitol. *See* Sugar.

THICKENERS Absorb water in foods, keep compounds mixed.

	NATURAL	
Alginate Propylene Glycol Alginate	Dairy Products Frostings Candy Beer Sodas	Safe
Carrageenan	Ice Cream Chocolate Milk Jelly	Small Amounts Safe Large Amounts Can Harm Colon
Casein Sodium Caseinate	Ice Cream Sherbet Creamers	Beneficial
Corn Syrup	Candies Syrups Snack Foods Imitation Dairy	Empty Calories Tooth Decay
Gelatin	Dessert Mixes Dairy Products Beverages	Safe

ADDITIVES. WHAT TO LOOK FOR ON FOOD LABELS

Gums Arabic Funcelleran Ghatti Guar Locust Bean Tragacanth	Ice Cream Puddings Salad Dressings Dough Cottage Cheese Candy Drink Mixes Fast Food Burgers	Poorly Tested
Sodium Carboxmethyl- cellulose	Ice Cream Pie Fillings Icings Diet Foods Candy Beer	Safe
Sorbitol	Diet Drinks Diet Foods Coconut Candy Gum	Safe Doesn't Raise Blood Sugar As Fast As Other Sugars
Starch Modified Starch	Soups Gravies	Safe

ADRENALINE The stress hormone. Increased adrenaline causes your system to speed up, and that includes your metabolism. While this may seem like a good thing to a dieter who wants a faster metabolism, the after-effects are not. Stress causes nutrient depletion, and anxiety that leads to eating (for dieters). One of the major causes of overeating is stress. *See* Stress.

▲ **AFFIRMATIONS** Positive self-statements. This is a behavior technique to change the way you view yourself and the world. Essentially it means re-thinking and re-phrasing the negative statements you make to yourself, in order to gain a more positive framework for succeeding with weight loss and lifestyle change. For instance, you might say: "I never do anything right." While you might mean this in good humor, or you might think you don't seriously believe this, by saying it, you are making a judgment about yourself. To be self-affirmative, you don't have to go to the opposite extreme and say: "I do everything right." You want to think of the things you did right and succeeded with in the past, and call them to mind when you doubt your own abilities or put yourself down verbally. If you only see the mistakes in your efforts, you need to shift your point of view to find the value in your efforts. It's there. You just have to look. When you're dealing with food and eating, rather than look at what you can't do, the self-affirming position would be to look at what you can do. *See* Rationalizations and Mirror Exercises for examples.

● **ALCOHOL** A depressant with calories. Alcohol is a double-edged sword. The first drink acts as a stimulant, making you feel relaxed and more outgoing. The second drink acts as a depressant, slowing your system down, dulling your reaction time. Alcohol withdraws water from your tissues and cells. In excess, this destroys brain cells. A low amount of alcohol can be neutralized by your liver, but when you have food in your stomach, your liver can only neutralize one drink per hour. If you drink too much alcohol, your liver adapts by increasing its tolerance, but it becomes fatty, and in severe cases, scarred. Two drinks per week is considered safe for a dieter, but not the sweet ones. A glass of wine every other day will not create problems. But you have to watch out! Alcohol dulls your senses and you forget that you're dieting. The foods you reach for when you're drinking alcohol are usually sugars, fats, and salts.

▲ **ALL OR NOTHING THINKING** A behavior term for thinking in extremes. Also called black and white thinking, either/or thinking. To a dieter, this means: either you are on a diet feeling deprived of all pleasure, or you are off a diet giving in to food whims telling yourself you'll start another diet next month. This pattern of thinking is failure-bound. It's based on negative input for both extremes – or lose/lose (everything but fat). When you're not on a diet, you feel guilty and critical of yourself. When you're on a diet, you want fast results to make up for lost time. You get disappointed easily if a diet doesn't provide major weight loss right away. This is a difficult mindset to maintain, because it provides you little personal pleasure and keeps your head-war going about weight.

To change this pattern, you must first change the way you perceive a diet. A diet isn't a short-term affair where you can starve yourself to ideal body weight, then somehow magically maintain it. Successful dieting is a gradual *process* where you earn leanness through sound nutrition, using behavior skills to change weight-gaining habits into supportive lean ones. You can change an all-or-nothing approach to food by learning moderation – eating smaller portions of a wide variety of foods, and substituting low-fat foods for their high-fat equivalents. In this way, you avoid the 'good food/bad food' extremes regarding your body's fuel. One dish of ice cream won't add pounds of fat, but a dish every night will add weight over time. When you deal with your food and eating attitudes from a more moderate perspective, you steadily ingrain less extreme patterns you need to get lean and stay lean. The positive effect flows over into other decision making areas of your life.

● **AMINO ACIDS** Nutrient components of protein. Approximately 22 amino acids occur in protein foods, in different combinations. They are broken down in your body to make other combinations. Your body can manufacture some of its own amino acids, but it cannot make 8 of the amino acids. These are called essential, since you must get them from your food. The 8 essential amino acids are: isoleucine, leucine, lysine, methionine, phenylalanine, threonine, tryptophan, and valine. You wouldn't need this list of essential amino acids, if it were not for tryptophan and phenylalanine, more commonly known amino acids. Phenylalanine is often used as an ingredient in diet aids or so-called "magic pill" formulas sold in magazines as a cure for weight. Tryptophan was used as a sleeping aid, until it was linked to a rare blood disease. It's important to realize that your amino acids must be provided in the right proportions for your body to use them. If they are not, it can throw off your metabolism of protein. Taking any amino acid in isolation is not a healthy idea, and one you should beware. *See* Tryptophan. Protein.

ANOREXIA NERVOSA An eating disorder characterized by reduction of food intake to the point of self-starvation.

Anorexia is a chronic condition that requires medical intervention, and often hospitalization. It is easily recognizable as excessive thinness to an emaciated state, or loss of at least 1/4 of normal weight. The individual is malnourished, and usually refuses to maintain normal weight. Severe losses of muscle mass become life threatening. Other complications include: breast atrophy, thin hair, dry skin, edema of legs, a layer of fine hair over the body, intolerance to cold, slow heart rate, low blood pressure to the degree of dizziness, menstrual disturbances, abdominal pain and bloating.

Anorexia is particularly difficult because the individual usually resists treatment and is reluctant to enter therapy. The disorder involves unresolved family conflicts making the person feel powerless in their own life. Control is exercised over food and the body as a way to feel power.

Treatment is long-term and includes dealing with nutritional deficiencies, medical conditions, body image distortions, assertiveness behavior, and exercise patterns.

If you, or anyone you know, suffers from this disease, don't feel that it can be resolved with an at home plan, or a change in diet. Find medical help without delay, for life's sake.

ANTHROPOMETRIC MEASUREMENTS Traditional tests to determine body fat and muscle composition. Clinical pinch-an-inch. Anthropometrics takes into account weight, height, mid-upper arm circumference, skin-fold thickness in the triceps, and mid-upper arm muscle circumference. The measuring device for skinfold thickness is the caliper, which resembles a large metal pincher or tweezers. The mid-upper arm muscle circumference is an indirect result of the other tests, and is based on hundreds of clinical averages, using a formula to arrive at this number. The tests measure subcutaneous fat tissue. *See* Scale, for the recommended levels of healthy body fat content.

▲ **ANXIETY** Fear or uncertainty about the future. *See* Relaxation to let it go.

APPETITE Your body's internal nutrient regulator, with cues for hunger and satiety. Your appetite originates in your brain, in the hypothalamus. Both aspects of eating are controlled there, hunger and satiety. Various chemicals stimulate this area, creating hunger pangs or the urge to eat, and ending hunger with fullness or a chemical cue for nutrient satisfaction. Scientists are not sure of the exact causes for hunger and satiety, or exactly what triggers the process. However, they have identified some of the key chemicals that are involved.

Glucose is an important factor in hunger. When blood glucose is low, the cue to eat is signalled. Glucose is the nutrient from carbohydrates, derived in the digestive process. It's the primary source of energy for your muscles and brain. Scientists believe that the brain contains a glucose receptor, a gauge for blood levels. When glucose levels rise, from eating carbohydrates, the cue to stop eating is given. An easy way to stop hunger would be to eat complex carbohydrates. They're low-fat, satisfying, and fibrous. Carbohydrate snacks during the day would keep glucose levels stable.

Insulin is another important factor in hunger and satiety. But it's also related to glucose too. When glucose levels are high in your blood, insulin is released. According to researcher Judith Wurtman, the insulin increases the amount of tryptophan that goes to your brain. Tryptophan stimulates the production of serotonin, a neurotransmitter in your brain. Serotonin turns off hunger.

Neurotransmitters are brain chemicals that transmit messages through your nerves and to your muscles. When your brain has high levels of the neurotransmitters serotonin, norepinephrine, epinephrine and dopamine, appetite is reduced. Exercise increases the production of epinephrine and norepinephrine. Stress on your body, such as exercise lead to an increase in the neurotransmitters. This is one of the reasons why exercise is an excellent substitute for eating.

Cholecystokinin is a hormone in your small intestines, produced after eating. Researchers believe that it can act on the hypothalamus to produce satiety.

Fiber has been credited with a decrease in hunger, by creating fullness in the stomach. But many researches feel that the stomach has no direct effect on hunger or satiety. Rather, the stomach fullness creates a sense of satisfaction, or a feeling of fullness, which causes the individual to stop eating. Fiber is also a component of carbohydrates. So it all might go back to glucose again.

The biochemical factors in hunger are only part of the picture. People eat for many reasons, even when they don't feel hungry. Regulating these hungers falls into the domain of habit control, and taking charge of the emotional appetite. *See* Hunger, Psychological. Habits.

APPETITE SUPPRESSANTS

DRUGS Anorectic agents that chemically reduce hunger. Many experts say that amphetamine-type agents (but not amphetamines) can be helpful in the early stages of a diet, particularly for people who have severe hunger problems and a history of diet failure. But they recommend that these agents only be used for the first 2-3 months in conjunction with a sound diet and exercise program, and only in the care of your doctor.

The downside of appetite suppressants involves more than the stated risks or side effects. While these chemicals do not *directly* cause nutritional imbalance, they can lead to it, because of what they do – suppress your natural appetite. Your appetite is the regulator of your nutrient needs. Without it, you won't get a reading on nutritional depletion. When your appetite is suppressed, you may not eat balanced meals, you may eat very little, or nothing at all, thinking less food is better, less food will let you lose weight faster. This can result in the opposite effect you were striving for – inferior weight loss caused by muscle wasting, and inferior health brought on by nutrient deficiency. This will cause weight regain.

While a chemical may be judged safe, this safety exists in isolation, not in the user's framework. The users of appetite suppressants are people with weight problems

– and that means habit problems – often addictive food habits. This is the most likely person to become emotionally dependent on the pills, or overuse them. Many dieters misuse the pills, thinking more is better regardless of the recommended dose. It's like getting a free credit card in the mail, when you have a habit of over-extending.

The best course is to forget the pills, and use a sound diet and exercise program alone. That way, you get the results without risks. The list below shows you some of the most common chemical agents used to curb appetites. Many of them are the main ingredient in over-the-counter aids you can get without a prescription. Always check with your doctor before using any chemical aid or adjunct to your diet to be on the safe side. After the list of chemical suppressors, we've developed a list of *natural* appetite suppressors that are your body's best defense against weight problems. You can weigh the difference.

APPETITE-SUPPRESSING CHEMICALS

Amphetamines. They're prescription anorectic agents which stimulate your nervous system. They were widely-used for weight loss years ago, until the side effects were catalogued. These include: nervousness, irritability, insomnia, blurred vision, dizziness, palpatations, sweating, nausea, vomiting, and sometimes hypertension. They also lead to dependency. They stimulate your hypothalamus (brain center for appetite), which decreases your appetite. They are now prohibited in many states for use in weight control.

Phenylpropanolamine (PPA).This is the ingredient in most over-the counter appetite suppressants. It's chemically related to amphetamine, and stimulates your central nervous system, but in a lower degree. The side effects include nervousness, insomnia, headaches, nausea, and tinnitus (ringing in your ears). They stimulate your hypothalamus, which decreases your appetite. You should check with your doctor before using PPA. NOT FOR USE BY PEOPLE WITH HIGH BLOOD PRESSURE, THYROID, KIDNEY OR HEART DISEASE. You don't need to risk side effects like these for weight loss.

Benzocaine. This is the ingredient in most over-the-counter candies, lozenges and gums for weight control. It's a topical anesthetic that numbs your tongue, reducing your ability to taste food. It's presumed that if you can't taste food, you won't desire it as much, or eat as much. This could mean that you become nutrient-deficient, because you're not eating. Or it can have the opposite effect than intended. You eat more high-sweet foods, without realizing how sweet and fattening they are.

Methylcellulose. This is the ingredient in bulkers, such as fiber tablets, laxatives and fiber cookies. It absorbs liquid in your stomach, creating a feeling of fullness. It can absorb up to 50 times its weight. There's no harm in these adjuncts, providing that you eat a balanced diet simultaneously and take a vitamin/mineral supplement, since you can suffer loss of minerals. But be sure to check for sodium content. Don't see these as a cure for weight gain, or rely on them for a major part of your day, since they are only aids. Never use them instead of *food, since that will lead to muscle losses, which causes fat gain.*

NATURAL APPETITE SUPPRESSANTS

Cholecystokinin. This is a hormone that is produced in your intestines after you eat. It stimulates your hypothalamus, which suppresses hunger. If you eat lean, you get your hunger suppressed and excellent fat burn, with NO RISKS.

Glucose. This is the nutrient created from digestion of carbohydrates. When it reaches your brain, hunger is terminated. When your daily diet is high in complex-carbohydrates, your hunger is naturally abated all day.

And you get the double benefits of better fat burn, with NO RISKS. If you eat your snacks as carbohydrates, you can have your hunger terminated, along with a boost of natural energy.

Insulin. This is the hormone produced by your pancreas to regulate your glucose metabolism. It increases the amount of tryptophan that gets to your brain, which in turn, produces a neurotransmitter called serotonin, which turns off your hunger. This is a natural part of digestion of carbohydrates.

Exercise. Sustained aerobic activity produces endorphines, which are neurotransmitters in your brain that stimulate your hypothalamus to turn off hunger. One aerobic workout also depletes your body's carbohydrate stores, so your ready for another carbohydrate boost, which will turn off hunger again.

The cycle of healthy eating and regular exercise is the best appetite suppressant you can find. *See* Appetite.

ARTIFICIAL SWEETENERS Imitation sugar. Aspartame, saccharin, cyclamates. Of the three synthetic sweeteners, only aspartame is considered safe so far, and is still being tested. The others are linked to cancer. There is an issue you should consider regarding aspartame. Since it contains a synthetic version of one of the essential amino acids, phenylalanine, and since the amino acids must be balanced to work properly, excessive use of one amino acid, without the presence of the others, doesn't suggest safety. Studies indicate that imbalanced amino acids can inhibit protein synthesis by your body. Until more is known about the intricate workings of the amino acids in tandem and in isolation, it's best to play it safe. When in doubt, do without. The calories you save by using artificial sweeteners can be saved a better way, by cutting fats. *See* Sugar.

ARTERIOSCLEROSIS Cholesterol buildup in artery walls. Also called hardening of the arteries, because the arteries harden with the plaque deposits. *See* Cholesterol.

● **ASSERTIVENESS** The ability to act definitively in your own behalf. Many diets talk about assertiveness as the ability to say No — to food that makes you fat, to habits that promote fat, and often, they mean say NO to foods and habits that aren't on the *particular* diet plan. You've got to be very careful about the choice you make for weight loss, because assertiveness is really about *choosing for yourself.* Lack of assertiveness is generally associated with overweight and obesity. A combination of improper eating and lack of exercise, along with a number of environmental and emotional factors cause weight gain. And once weight is gained, you become less assertive.

What does that actually mean? Does that mean you can't be trusted with food? Does it mean you can't be trusted to stand up for yourself in situations where food is involved? If you choose a diet that makes those choices for you, giving you lists and rules, and only certain foods you can eat, are you learning to be assertive?

One of the primary keys to being assertive is to *know* what you want and need. That's not as easy as it sounds. Many people don't take enough time to explore their *real* needs and feelings, let alone express them. Non-assertive people tend to let everyone else express their needs, and they also tend to try to help everyone else with their problems, leaving little time for themselves.

If that sounds like you, you might buy a small pocket notebook, and begin to jot down feelings you have about yourself, and needs you have that don't seem to be met. It's like a diary — but it's not about someone else, it's about you. This diary is for you to think about your needs, it doesn't mean you have to confront people about your needs. Your diary can start with cues like:

"I like ________________" Make a list of the things you like and give yourself more of them.

"I need ________________" Make a list of the things you need and think about how to meet those needs.

"I was confused by ________________" If a situation makes you feel put down or ineffective, describe what it was and what came about to make you feel that way. Then do a few mental rehearsals to set that situation up again in your mind, and resolve it in a way that would make you feel good. You'll find examples of mental rehearsals in the topic Relaxation.

Assertiveness is acting definitively for you. That also means acting positively for you. Your choice of a diet is far more important than dieting itself, when it comes to being assertive. Wanting to lose weight is a decision. Wanting to lose weight *effectively* is an assertive decision.

EFFECTIVE WEIGHT LOSS AND MAINTENANCE

How do you make a self-supportive diet and health decision? Choose safe weight loss, because that's the kind that's effective for both weight loss and maintenance.

1. Your weight loss should be slow and steady.
2. The best choice is real food.
3. The program should fit into your lifestyle, so you'll keep doing it. That means you have to ask yourself who you are, how you live and what you can live with. (And you should expect to live better, because of a diet, not worse, after it.)
4. Go for the maximum, not the minimum.
   The MINIMUM is weight loss at any price.
   The MAXIMUM is weight loss with pleasure.
   The MAXIMUM is a healthy, balanced diet, plus exercise, plus self-enrichment.

Lack of assertiveness is choosing NOT TO CHOOSE. Letting choices be made for you — doing what other people think is best for you. This year, choose yourself. Choose to concentrate on what you CAN DO, not what you CAN'T DO. Say YES to yourself. You have far more power over everything when you take it.

b

◆ **BASEBALL** Skill sport exercise, non-aerobic. *See* Exercise.

◆ **BASKETBALL** Skill sport aerobic exercise (if you keep moving) *See* Exercise.

▲ **BEHAVIOR MODIFICATION** The science of self-enhancement. Behavior Modification is a branch of psychology, but it differs from clinical psychology in its approach to problem-solving. While psychology goes after deep-seated causes for problems, in childhood and past experiences, behavior tackles problems in the present, as they express themselves in your attitudes and responses to situations. It is based on changing the things you *can* change, instead of dwelling on things you can't change, such as the past. For instance, if your response to a family crisis is to eat and feel guilty, you may not be able to change your family or the cause of the crisis, but you can change how you react to it. You can do relaxation exercises or go for a walk instead of eating. Both of these skills help you handle stress better, and help you stay more centered in crisis.

More than 100 clinical tests have demonstrated the effectiveness of behavior modification for weight control and maintenance. *See* all Behavior topics ▲.

● **BEVERAGES** Thirst quenchers. The following beverages are listed in the order that provides the most value to a dieter.

1. WATER. Necessary nutrient, no calories (includes water spritzers).
2. LOW FAT MILK DRINKS. Essential for calcium, excellent source of vitamins, minerals, low-calorie.
3. FRESH VEGETABLE JUICES. (Canned have too much salt). Excellent sources of vitamins, minerals and essential nutrients, low calorie.
4. FRESH FRUIT JUICES. (Watch out for sugar in bottled and canned versions). Excellent sources of vitamins/minerals and essential nutrients, low-calorie.
5. HERBAL TEAS. No nutrition, but positive therapeutic benefits.
6. CLUB SODA. No nutrition, but low-or-no calories. (Includes club soda spritzers – lime, lemon, cranberry. The fruits add a bit of nutrition.)
7. COFFEE. No nutrients, caffeine, water.
8. TEA. A tad of flouride, tannin, caffeine, oils.
9. FRUIT FLAVORED DRINKS. High calorie, high sugar.
10. CARBONATED SOFT DRINKS. High sugar, contain acids to keep sugar in suspension.
11. COLAS. 100% sugar, caffeine, additives.
12. DIET SODAS. Artificial sugars, additives.
13. ALCOHOL. Calories, mood changers.

◆ **BICYCLING (STATIONARY)** An aerobic exercise.

Benefits:

- Great cardiovascular training.
- Excellent calorie-burning exercise, if you pedal at sufficient speed and tension.
- Easy to use with minimal instruction.
- Easily exchanged with outdoor bicycle fun.
- Strengthens leg and back muscles.
- Readily available at most health spas.

- Very appropriate exercise for advanced pregnancy since the extra "baby weight" is not a prohibiting factor when sitting on a bike.
- Advanced technology, with computerized Lifecycles and fan bicycles (Airdyne), adds another dimension of challenge. (*Lifestyles* are computerized cycles, incorporating an interval-training workout, that enable you to individually program pace, duration, and degree of difficulty along any desired incline. *Fan Cycles,* which are relatively uncommon on the health spa scene, have long arm bars that move up and back as you pedal, giving you an upper-body workout as well. In addition, the front wheel of the bicycle has a fan generated by pedaling, to keep you cooled off as you work out.)

Guidelines:
To properly adjust your seat height to avoid leg cramps, knee strain, and leg fatigue:

- Sit on the seat and rotate the right pedal to the down position.
- Place the ball of your foot on the pedal. Your leg should be fully extended. Test for a slight knee bend rather than a knee lock and adjust the height of the seat.

If you cycle outdoors with a conventional bicycle:

- Use a standard bicycle or adjust the gears on your ten speed to pedal with some tension.
- Keep your speed comfortable and steady. Avoid too much gliding when the bike is working without you.
- Invest in safety gear such as a helmet, reflectors, rear view mirror, lights, and reflective clothing for night riding.

BILE An enzyme produced by your liver, used in digestion to break up fats. *See* Digestion.

▲ **BINGE** A bout of excessive eating. To dieters, this usually means breaking a diet by eating foods not listed on the plan — cheating eating. Or eating anything you want for a period of time away from your diet, especially sweets and fats. In some cases, such as during starvation diets, binges occur because your body cannot sustain itself on low–or–no nutrition, and the binge provides needed energy. Many very low calorie diets have been known to provoke cycles of binging, because of lack of adequate nutrition.

In non-starvation situations, binges occur because you *want* something you feel you can't have, such as chocolate cake. This is common to dieters who have good food/bad food divisions in their minds, and the pattern needs to be modified with behavior education. If you believe you will never be allowed to eat chocolate cake again, the likelihood of a binge on chocolate is greater. But when you realize you can eat chocolate cake again, but eat less of it, and find low fat versions, the pressure of forced deprivation is released. While binge eating can be biochemical in origin or emotional, it is an unhealthy eating practice that can escalate if it is not dealt with and moderated. The term *binge,* used by dieters is a borrowed word that comes from a more serious eating disorder and should not be confused with the binge common to Bulimia. See Break.

BINGE/PURGE SYNDROME Eating and vomiting or taking laxatives, or both. *See* Bulimia.

▲ **BLAME** Finding fault, usually in yourself. A self-critical habit pattern. *See* Relaxation to let it go.

BLOOD PRESSURE The cardiac output of your heart — stroke and volume. Good blood pressure is systolic below 140, and diastolic below 90, or below 140/90. To reduce your blood pressure, reduce your sodium and fat, eat more fiber, exercise and don't smoke.

BODY COMPOSITION The nutrient structure of your body. A healthy body at ideal weight has approximately the follow composition:

WATER	55%
PROTEIN(BODY MUSCLE TISSUE)	20%
FAT	15-20%
CARBOHYDRATES	2%
MINERALS	2%
VITAMINS	LESS THAN 1%

If you have more fat, you have less muscle. The rest should remain stable. You have to replace your water, vitamins, minerals, carbohydrates, and protein daily. But if you have extra fat, you don't need to include much fat in your diet.

BODY IMAGE How you see yourself. *See* Mirror Exercises. Imagery, for a healthy body image.

BODY TYPE Your genetic shape, form and composition. Physique.

There are three primary body types that can be determined by clear, observable features. These types were identified from classification of athletes for sports participation. ECTOMORPH linear. Symbolized by column. MESOMORPH broad shouldered. Symbolized by inverse triange. ENDOMORPH round all over. Symbolized by circle.

One of the biggest mistakes people make is moving out of their body type for their weight loss goal. This causes two basic problems: you can't reach your goal and remain dis-satisfied, and you don't take advantage of the potential within your body type. When you learn to appreciate your own unique body type and work within its limits and capacities, you gain a better body image and have more realistic goals for fitness.

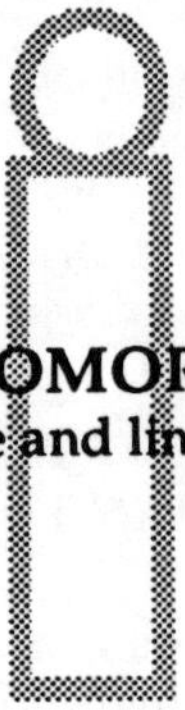

ECTOMORPH
lithe and linear

- Small boned
- Long arms,legs
- Shoulder to Hip Line is similar
- Low muscle, low fat
- Lithe bodies
- Can eat more without gaining weight

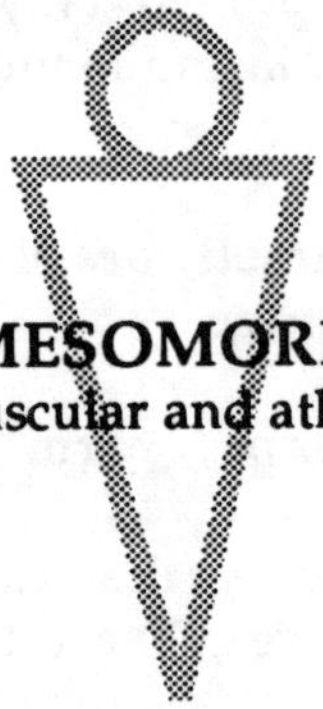

MESOMORPH
muscular and athletic

- Denser boned
- Average length arms, legs
- Shoulder to Hip Line narrows in at hips
- High muscle, medium fat
- Athletic bodies
- Lose weight and gain muscle easier

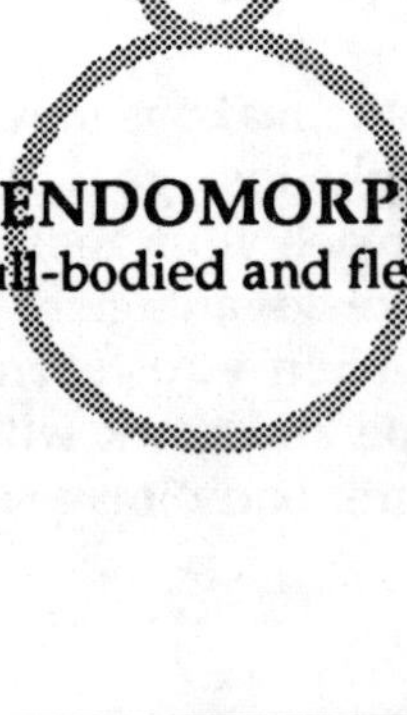

ENDOMORPH
full-bodied and fleshy

- Medium boned
- Short arms, legs
- Shoulder to Hip Line is similar from wider hips
- Low muscle, high fat
- Round large bodies
- Have the most difficulty with weight loss

How To Optimize Your Body Type

Ectomorphic men and women who want more upper body differentiation can build upper body muscles with weight lifting or swimming.

Mesomorphic men and women have the best results with weight loss, due to their innately high muscular content. However, women who don't want to appear too broad shouldered and muscular, should avoid weight lifting, or use it with low weights and lots of reps, rather than high weights, since mesomorphs have a tendency to build up fast. This must be combined with a low fat diet that is carbohydrate rich, and balanced in protein, so that muscles aren't pumped up under a layer of fat. Stretching and limbering exercises are excellent for mesomorphs, especially men, to avoid that bulky, non-flexible look that can develop with weight lifting.

Endomorphic men and women have the most trouble losing weight, because of their innately high body fat content. However, endomorphic women are known for their hourglass figures, and can carry more fat without it making their bodies look off balance. (Example: Marilyn Monroe.) Endomorphic people should guard their fat intake on a regular basis to avoid excess fat. Rapid weight loss diets are the least preferred method for endomorphs who can regain more rapidly than an ectomorph or mesomorph (who have more body muscle). Full body aerobic workouts are most beneficial to endomorphs, along with stretches for muscle lengthening, so the overall appearance is longer, rather than rounder. This body type is best served by staying on a diet a little longer, to insure that the ideal weight you reach is stabilized by higher body muscle content inside. This is also the body type that needs regular exercise to keep weight gain away, but the results are worth it. Your efforts are more noticeable, since fat loss really shows, and this incentive can outweigh the fact that it's more difficult for you to lose weight.

Most people fall midway on the line between body types, and all types can share common fat distribution tendencies. *See* Fat Distribution.

BODY WEIGHT Water, muscle and fat. *See* Weight.

● **BREADS** Grains. A food in the grain group for essential nutrition. The processed breads with white flour and added sugar and fat don't really qualify as real grains. They're fats in grain suits. The whole grain breads are the better sources, as low in sugar and fat as you can find them. *See* Grains. Food Groups.

▲ **BREAK** A lapse in dieting. A guilt state for hard-core dieters. Fear of breaking your diet is more common on rapid weight lose diets that presume you have to lose weight by a certain date, and you won't lose it if you eat foods that are not on the program. If you are on a natural diet plan, where you are eating leaner foods with a wide variety of options, a break doesn't mean disaster or doom.

Guilt comes into play when you have abnormal food views built into the diet — you have your foods, and the other foods aren't good for you. When you see food from this perspective of good and bad, can't have and can, then the odds are greater that you'll long for the ones you aren't allowed. If you see food in a broader perspective, as energy to moderate for weight loss, you don't feel as deprived, and you can take a break without feeling guilty about it.

This doesn't mean that you can lose weight even if you eat anything you want. It means you understand the challenge you are undertaking with food moderation and weight loss. You don't need to spend energy on guilt and self-recrimination. They aren't feelings that move you forward. They can set you back. In fact, they can make you eat. Often, people break diets for very substantial reasons:

1. The diet is too restrictive. Regimented eating and narrowly-focused eating plans can create diet stress and head-wars about food. After a few weeks of feeling ostracized from the real world, you might need a break.
2. Your nutritional needs aren't being met. If you are on a diet that does not provide your essential nutrients, you will be hungry constantly, and you will break your diet. In this case, it is beneficial. Getting nutrients in a diet lapse is your body's way of protecting itself.

Of course, most dieters don't go for nutrition when they break a diet. They go for sugar or fat. This is part of the reward/punishment principle that is inherent in rigid diets. After you spend three weeks without a sweet on a rigid plan, you feel punished for having a weight problem. To reward yourself, you eat something they won't allow, a food that made you feel good in the past. It's the double-edged sword of deprived diets. You can spend most of your time on a deprived diet feeling like a child who was sent to your room without dessert because you were bad. Some programs even use childish language that enhances your sense of guilt: "You didn't lose weight this week. You were a bad girl/boy."

Some dieters like this kind of feedback and feel it keeps them on track. But it doesn't mix well with the rest of your life. That same guilty child who was bad for not losing weight this week, has to go to the office, and lock up a big business deal, then go home and feel he or she can't be trusted to make decisions about food. Does that sound familiar to you? Does it sound logical or self-supportive?

If you're tired of guilt, and don't need more, try a healthy food plan where you make your own choices. Realize that you will make a few good decisions and you'll make a few bad ones, and keep re-training yourself to make the good ones. That's personal power.

➠ How To Manage A Diet Break

If you are on a diet, and you have a piece of cake, or eat half the contents of the refrigerator, handle it logically.

1. Write down what you ate and tally the fat, sugar, and calories.
2. Decide which energy you wanted, the fat or the sugar, or maybe the salt. Jot down your feelings about what you ate. Take as long as you want. Draw cartoons if it pleases you.
3. Go for a walk, or do a relaxation exercise to ease your stress.
4. Identify non-fattening foods you can substitute for the foods you ate, and have them on hand in case you feel yourself wanting to break again.
5. Begin again the next day.

If you break your diet again, follow the same plan. As long as you keep the majority of your week intact with lean choices and regular exercise, you won't put on a pound of fat from a break. Keep trying to resolve your food issues, without guilt or blame. That's the nature of healthy eating, and healthy weight loss.

● **BREAKFAST** The first source of energy in your day. This is one of the most important meals for a dieter. If you skip it, you miss the metabolic benefits, since your metabolism comes out of sleep, burning at a lower rate. The introduction of food in the morning starts the production of heat, and kicks off an active metabolism early in the day. This keeps you on an even keel all day, burning fat at a steady pace. The less fat you eat in the morning, the better off you will be, and there are many breakfast fares that are high carbohydrate and low fat. Cereal, milk and fruit. A whole wheat waffle with strawberries. A toasted bagel with jelly and a piece of fruit. Breakfast is also important to insure that you get your calcium. Don't skip it, thinking you'll lose weight faster. You'll burn fat better when you eat breakfast.

▲ **BREATHING** A gas-exchange process where oxygen is supplied to your blood on inhaling, and carbon-dioxide wastes are released by exhaling. Since oxygen is mandatory to all life processes, breathing is often synonymous with life, and your oxygen uptake a barometer of that life. Better oxygen uptake means better health, heart, circulation, digestion, metabolism, cell regeneration and repair. Dieters should note that oxygen is needed for fat burn, and to enhance that, you need to improve your breathing capacity.

The two basic types of breathing are chest breathing (shallow breathing) and diaphragm breathing (deep breathing). Babies breathe from their diaphragms as nature intended, while adults tend to fall into the habit of chest breathing, and need breathing re-training to take up more oxygen.

The goals of breathing exercises are:

1. To increase your breathing awareness – how you are currently breathing as opposed to how you should be breathing.
2. To expand your breath capacity, in order to increase your oxygen uptake. This will energize your body, relax your mind, and improve your overall health.
3. To provide an instant relaxation technique you can use in times of stress.

The benefits of proper breathing are immediate, and you don't need special equipment, clothing, or location. You can do it without interrupting other work. At first, you should practice at home alone to learn the techniques, then you can carry them over to other activities and sports. An especially good combination is walking while using deep breathing techniques.

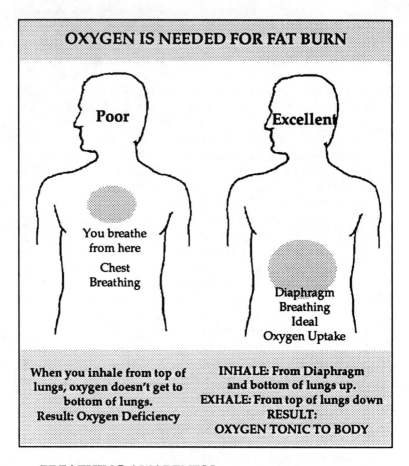

OXYGEN IS NEEDED FOR FAT BURN

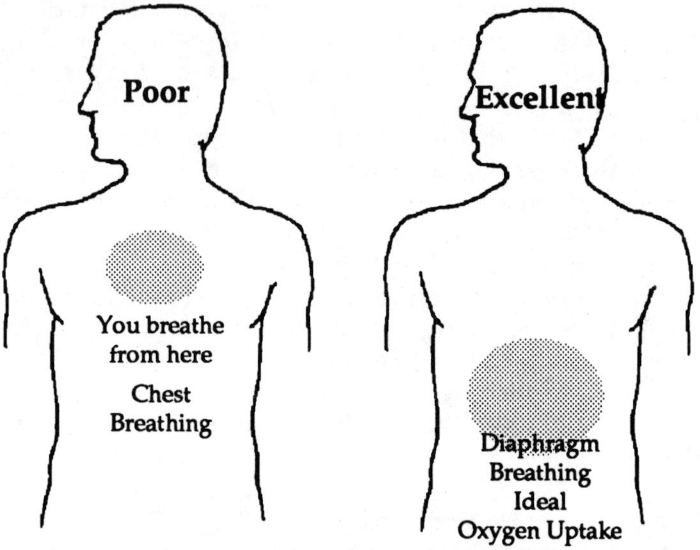

**When you inhale from top of lungs, oxygen doesn't get to bottom of lungs.
Result: Oxygen Deficiency**

**INHALE: From Diaphragm and bottom of lungs up.
EXHALE: From top of lungs down
RESULT:
OXYGEN TONIC TO BODY**

BREATHING AWARENESS

➠ **How To Improve Your Breathing**

Sit in a comfortable chair and breathe normally for 5 minutes. Notice whether you breathe from your upper chest or deeply into your abdomen. In chest breathing, you would be inhaling from your upper lungs and your shoulders would tend to rise up. In diaphragm breathing, you would be inhaling from your lower lungs, and your

CHEST BREATHING	DIAPHRAGM BREATHING
half breathing	whole breathing deep breathing
Decreases oxygen uptake by limiting the amount of air that reaches your lower lungs	Increases oxygen uptake by pulling air into lower portion of your lungs where most of your blood circulates. This makes more oxygen available to your blood
Puts strain on your heart, making it pump more blood. Blood has to circulate faster to carry available oxygen. This means higher blood pressure	Lowers blood pressure Reduces heart rate Reduces stress on heart
Associated with anxiety Related to stress breathing and its accompanying symptoms	Associated with calmness Increases production of endorphines — natural opiates

abdomen would balloon out, then your ribs would rise up, then your lungs would fill with air. Practice deep breathing for 5 minutes and compare the two experiences.

Deep Breathing. Sit in a comfortable chair with your feet flat on the floor and your back straight, in order to free up your diaphragm. Regulate your breathing process for 10 minutes. Breathe in and out through your nostrils down to your abdomen to the following count:

Inhale while counting slowly to 3
Exhale while counting slowly to 3

Your goal is to make the inhale and exhale match. You can increase your breathing capacity by increasing the count, as it becomes more comfortable. If you find yourself getting dizzy or hyperventilating, you can prevent this by alternating your breaths between shallow and deep. Practice this technique until it becomes like second nature.

Breathing Expertise. Sit in a comfortable chair with your feet flat on the floor and your back straight. Regulate your diaphragm breathing to this count:

Inhale while counting slowly to 3
Exhale while counting slowly to 6

Many experts feel that this style of breathing creates the best benefits. The exhale length is double the time for inhaling. You will feel the difference immediately.

BREATHING HINTS:

- Never strain. Never try to force air into your lungs.
- Keep your mind blank by concentrating on the breathing itself.
- Keep your mouth closed. It helps if you keep your tongue on the roof of your mouth.
- You can place your fingers lightly on your abdomen to insure that it is ballooning out, to show that you are breathing from your diaphragm.
- Keep your jaw relaxed.
- Wear loose, comfortable clothes that don't restrain your diaphragm.
- You can mildly contract your abdomen at the end of breathing to expel last stale air.
- You can vary your breathing with a holding count of 3, between inhaling and exhaling. This retains oxygen and enhances it's pickup.

➠ How To Use Your Breathing Expertise

Stressed and about to eat? Consciously switch to a pattern of deep breathing from your diaphragm. You will relax and feel in control.

Combine your breathing exercises with assertiveness statements, such as "In with health, out with fat," or "In with positive, out with negative." It will strengthen your inner resources.

Combine your breathing exercises with mental rehearsals for success, by creating stressful situations which can cause you to eat, and resolving them in your imagination. *See* Relaxation.

BROWN FAT A type of fat in your body that is viewed as "fat that keeps you lean." The primary site of brown fat is the upper back (identified in animals). It is more metabolically active than your standard white fat that is found in your adipose tissue. It is usually activated in cold climates to keep you from freezing. Brown fat may help to explain the "hot" feeling you get on upper back sometimes when you eat or exercise, but not enough research has been done on brown fat to clearly link it to obesity. Only 1% of your fat is brown fat, as opposed to white fat which can be 20-30% of your body weight. Since brown fat is active fat, and very little is stored in your body, it's not fat that you need to lose.

▲ **BUDDY SYSTEM** a next best friend for a dieter. An individual, group, or network of friends to support your weight loss efforts and be there when you need help. An ideal buddy would be a former dieter who succeeded, because no one understands the struggle to lose weight better than someone who has been through it. If your buddy is a current dieter, be sure you don't support each other's desire to let go and fall back into old habits. If you choose a buddy who is overweight and settled into it, what might that indicate about you? (A secret desire to stay overweight? Fear of failure?) If your buddy is a slim person who never had a weight problem, be sure that person has a genuine appreciation for health and fitness, not just image or appearance.

Try not to think of a diet counsellor or program representative as your buddy, because their role is an overseer, and their professional obligations to their own programs make it hard for them to be objective. Also, when you use your counsellor as a buddy, it's like handing your control over to someone else, and you want to avoid that. Many dieters find buddies in their families, but it's not the usual choice because of the emotional connections. It can put too much stress on family members and thwart your efforts. Part of taking control of your weight and health is "getting independent." It's difficult to get independent from a family member. Your diet buddy should not be someone who intimidates you, pressures you, or makes you feel uncomfortable in crisis. It should be someone who reinforces you, relaxes you, reminds you of your achievements, and guides you to make the right decisions, *not someone who makes decisions for you.* The reason your diet buddy isn't your best friend is simple. That role is waiting to be claimed by you.

You might say, "I don't know anyone who can be my buddy. I have no one to turn to." That's a very common problem, or we wouldn't have the weight problems we see today. Be creative about finding your buddy system. You can rely on your spiritual beliefs as a buddy system or you can acquire audio & video tapes for support. In a pinch, you can call Overeater's Anonymous. They're there for everyone.

BULIMIA An eating disorder characterized by bouts of overeating followed by self-induced vomiting, abuse of laxatives, diuretics or excessive exercise — for the purpose of weight control. Also called binge/purge syndrome. Literal meaning: ox hunger. High-carbohydrate (refined) foods are common binge choices. Often, no outward signs of the disorder seem observable, since most bulimics stay within normal weight ranges, and binge/purge secretly. Bulimia is a serious eating disturbance which requires professional evaluation and treatment with individual or group therapy combined with other disciplines such as behavior modification, nutritional counselling and medications.

The problem is of special concern to dieters because mild eating disorders can spiral out of control, and become major eating disorders, particularly after bouts of bad dieting. Bulimia frequently occurs in adolescents after rigid dieting. This raises concern for teenagers and college students who have been known to experiment with purging, and laxatives as forms of weight control.

The following list of problems common to bulimia is alarming because it reads like a profile of an average dieter:

1. Good Food/Bad Food Syndrome. Seeing diet foods as good foods and most other foods as bad foods.
2. Obsessive Concern with Slimness
3. Distorted Eating Patterns
4. Food Preoccupation
5. The Need for Rigid Diet Rules, often Self-Imposed
6. Body Image Disturbances — seeing yourself fatter than you are.
7. Shame, Guilt, Excessive Anxiety
8. Private Binging, often with fear of being unable to stop.
9. Difficulty Accepting Feelings. Tend to transfer feelings to food.
10. Distorted Thinking. Eating meals which results in full feeling or distended stomach, is equated with losing control over body weight.

The bulimic's problems are chronic versions of some of the issues that concern dieters. In the beginning stages of the disorder, purging and laxative use is voluntary, but as the disorder progresses, purging and laxative use become automatic, involuntary. A dieter may binge and feel guilty after eating 800-1000 calories, while a bulimic can eat 5,000-10,000 calories in one eating episode. This makes it even more important to educate younger people on the dangers of excessive eating and unrealistic weight control practices, and to act as role models for healthy behavior and nutrition habits. With social pressures for slimness and expectations for perfection mounting in our society, it's not difficult to see why eating disorders are escalating.

In its severe phases, bulimia can create electrolyte imbalances, irregular menstrual cycles, irregular heart rate and blood pressure, enlarged salivary glands, constipation, diarrhea and more dangerous symptoms such as cardiac rhythm abnormalities.

C

● **CAFFEINE** A central nervous system stimulant. Caffeine excess is similar to stress symptoms — increased respiration, pulse rate and blood pressure, you feel all revved up with no place to run, like the fight or flight response. When you are on a diet, it's best to limit your caffeine intake, since the effects will be more pronounced when you are eating fewer calories.

The maximum dose should be no more than 400 mg/day, but watch out for decaffeinated coffee as a substitute. The decaf that is water-processed is the safest kind. The other variety contains formaldehyde. Your best bet is to substitute water or juices for coffee or tea, instead of using decaf.

One of the benefits of caffeine is for asthmatics, since it speeds respiration, letting air in.

COMMON SOURCES OF CAFFEINE

Chocolate (Dark)	26 mg/bar
Chocolate (Milk)	10 mg/bar
Aspirins	32 mg/pill
Cold Preparations	30 mg/dose
Stimulants	100 mg/tablet
Antacids	32 mg/tablet
Pain Relievers	32-66 mg/pill
Cola	32-65 mg per can
Coffee Drip	85 mg/cup
Coffee Instant	60 mg/cup
Coffee Decaf	3 mg/cup
Tea Brewed	50 mg/cup
Tea Instant	30 mg/cup
Cocoa	6-14 mg/cup

● **CALCIUM** An essential mineral. The most important fact about calcium that you need to consider is the issue of absorption. Only about 20-30% of your daily intake is absorbed. This is one of the reasons why you should pay particular attention to your calcium intake, keeping at the maximum daily level in the lean choices. Lack of calcium can cause an increase in cholesterol, leading to calcium deposits in the arteries (arteriosclerosis). Lack of calcium can also lead to osteoporosis, particularly in women, who are a higher-risk group, because of hormonal changes in menopause which also accelerate calcium losses. When calcium levels are low in your bloodstream, and calcium is not provided in the daily food you eat, your body takes calcium from your bones and teeth. Bones usually store enough calcium to meet your body's needs, but when it doesn't come in through your diet, the losses are never restored to your bones. They lose density and become brittle, resulting in pain, loss of height, spinal deformities and easy fractures (osteoporosis).

Lack of calcium shows up in loose teeth, receding gums, infected gums, gingivitis, spasms in your muscles, severe menstrual cramps, and constant headaches.

THE GOOD NEWS IS, when you get 1200-1500/mg of Calcium each day, you can restore a good part of your bone density, have lower blood pressure, and gum problems will ease.It takes about six months, so today is the day to start insuring your calcium needs.

The best sources for absorption are low fat dairy products, low fat protein along with foods that contain phosphorous. The reason you want your calcium in a low-fat format is because calcium combines with fat in your intestines and it can be excreted instead of absorbed. The best way to take your calcium would be between meals, when you are not eating fat. Many experts recommend that you take 30% of your daily calcium before bed to insure absorption, and get the added benefit of a good night's sleep, since calcium is a sleep aid. It also protects against sunburn, prevents depression, regulates your heartbeat, and activates enzymes in metabolism.

Calcium metabolism occurs in the presence of Vitamins A,C,D and B Complex, along with the minerals phosphorous and potassium. If you are a chocolate eater, the oxalic acid can prevent calcium absorption. Smoking or taking Steroids can also lead to calcium deficiencies.

CALCIUM AT A GLANCE	
	RECOMMENDED DOSE — 800 MG/DAY WOMEN OVER 30 — 1000-2000 MG/DAY
AVOID	**RELY ON**
STEROIDS	Skim 300 mg
CHOCOLATE	Cottage Cheese 160 mg
	Low Fat Yogurt 360 mg
SMOKING	Green Leafy Vegetables
	Beans
FAT AND FATTY PROTEINS	Whole Grains
	Vitamin & Minerals
	Bonemeal Supplement 1/2 Tsp.
	DAILY EXERCISE

◆ **CALISTHENICS** Non-aerobic, rhythmic exercises for strength and endurance.

◆ **CALLANETICS** A stretching exercise routine that combines relaxation, breathing and stretching in one program. In addition to being an excellent form of muscle and spine elongation, the exercises tone, shape, and benefit well-being.

CALORIES Units of energy derived from food. Foods are grouped according to the nutrient energy (calories) they yield. There are only three nutrients that provide calories:

1 GRAM PROTEIN	4 CALORIES
1 GRAM CARBOHYDRATES	4 CALORIES
1 GRAM FAT	9 CALORIES

These three nutrients are essential to your body, for its growth, maintenance and repair. A healthy diet provides these nutrients in the proper proportions to meet your body's needs, without adding extra fat. Those proportions are:

PROTEIN 20% OF TOTAL CALORIES
CARBOHYDRATES 55-60% OF TOTAL CALORIES
FAT 20-25% OF TOTAL CALORIES

➡ How To Estimate Your Daily Calorie Needs

To estimate your daily calorie needs, use the following formula which is a weight maintenance formula — the amount of calories needed to maintain your *current* weight.

ACTIVE WOMEN	12-14 CALS PER POUND OF BODY WEIGHT
INACTIVE WOMEN	10-12 CALS PER POUND OF BODY WEIGHT

Smaller framed women use the lower number. Larger framed women use the higher number.

ACTIVE MEN	14-16 CALS PER POUND OF BODY WEIGHT
INACTIVE MEN	12-14 CALS PER POUND OF BODY WEIGHT

Smaller framed men use the lower number. Larger framed men use the higher number.

➠ **How To Determine Daily Calorie Needs For Dieting**

Use the same formula as above, EXCEPT you will use your *ideal body weight* (the weight you should be) for the weight. For instance, if you currently weigh 160 and should weigh 130, use the weight of 130, and multiply the calories/per pound of body weight to that number. In addition, USE THE INACTIVE CALORIE NUMBER to tally your diet calories, not the active one.

This will put you in the lean range of calories for dieting. EXAMPLE: Our 160 pound woman wants to weigh 130. She uses the inactive level of calories (10-12) to multiply with her ideal body weight (130). She comes up with a calorie range for her diet:

1300-1560 CALORIES PER DAY

If her ideal body weight should be 120, her calorie range would be:

1200-1440 CALORIES PER DAY

If she wanted to diet very seriously, she would use the lower number of calories for her daily calorie maximum. If she wanted to diet moderately, she would use the higher number of calories for her daily maximum.

◆ **CALORIE EXPENDITURE** Output. *See* Exercise.

● **CALORIE INTAKE** Input. *See* Food Groups.

● **CANDY** A source of sugar. *See* Sugar.

● **CARBOHYDRATES** The nutrient source of primary energy for your muscles and brain. Carbohydrates are your body's preferred source of energy and primary brain food. They are divided into two groups— simple (sugar) and complex (starches). Complex carbohydrates are long-chain simple sugars that are linked when you eat them and then split into simple sugars when your body digests and absorbs them. Why, then, are complex carbohydrates considered good and simple carbohydrates considered bad? The reason is found in the nutritional quality of the foods that contain these carbohydrates and your body's response to them.

First, complex carbohydrates are less-refined foods, and therefore are good sources of many naturally occurring nutrients. Simple carbohydrates, or sugars, are usually very refined foods that have been stripped of their naturally occurring nutrients. Second, your body has a slower, more natural response to eating complex carbohydrates, gradually breaking down the longer chain to use for energy over prolonged periods—a longer energy boost.

Complex carbohydrates start to be broken down earlier in digestion, with an enzyme in your saliva. They go through a longer process of digestion, and many experts feel that few carbohydrate calories ever get to fat storage. One aerobic workout can deplete your body's carbohydrate stores. The thermic effect of carbohydrates doesn't apply to the highly processed versions, because they usually have added fats and sugars and very little fiber. The fresh, natural sources are the best.

Sugars exist in a very simple form, which stimulates a very rapid insulin response. They are absorbed easily and leave you feeling hungry sooner than if you ate a complex carbohydrate — shorter energy boost. People who eat high-sugar diets get short bursts of energy and big, tired letdowns. The energy is not first-quality, and for fat loss, the simple sugars are self-defeating, since they usually occur in foods that also contain a lot of fat.

The starch group of complex carbohydrates includes grains and grain products as well as starchy vegetables such as corn. They are excellent sources of B vitamins and fiber, especially when whole-grain varieties are eaten.

Vegetables and fruits are often mentioned together, because they have similar nutrient compositions. While fruit contains natural simple sugar that makes it sweet and higher in calories than vegetables, both fruits and vegetables provide healthy supplies of fiber and essential nutrients such as Vitamins A and C. In fact, one fresh grapefruit and one medium carrot will satisfy your total daily requirements for Vitamins A and C.

◆ **CARDIOVASCULAR CONDITIONING** Using exercise to reach maximum oxygen uptake and target heart rate for best heart health.

Aerobic exercise improves the power of your heart and circulation. When activity is performed regularly and for sufficient periods of time, it can produce beneficial physiological changes. Your body becomes a better machine. It can take in, transport, and use oxygen at an increased rate. Your heart becomes a better pump, pushing more blood out with each stroke, and it rests longer between beats. Distribution and blood flow in your lungs and working muscles are enhanced, and slowing of your heart rate (pulse) occurs both at rest and at any given level of activity. As a result, your cardiovascular system operates more efficiently.

To achieve cardiovascular conditioning, certain conditions must be met:

- Duration: the exercise must be performed at a suitable level of intensity for 20 — 30 minutes (not counting warm-ups or cool-downs).
- Frequency: the exercise should be performed at least 3 times per week, preferably on alternate days.
- Intensity: the exercise must be strenuous enough for you to reach a level of exertion that is about 70 — 85 percent of your maximum heart rate.

The most suitable sports for cardiovascular conditioning are the ones that require repeated and continuous movement — running, swimming, cycling, brisk walking, rowing, rope skipping, running in place, stationary cycling, basketball, handball, racquetball, squash, skating, hockey, cross-country skiing, soccer, and hiking.

Other sports might not be adequate for cardiovascular conditioning if they allow long pauses between action or the movement takes place in brief spurts. In the same way that you want to keep the heat constant in your eating style, you need to keep the heat steady with your exercise. Low-heat exercises include baseball, softball, golf, and bowling.

Calisthenics that emphasize slow bending, stretching, and graceful movement will not provide cardiovascular benefits as well as continuous, rhythmic calisthenics that are performed at a higher level of intensity. *See* Exercise.

CAUSES (of overweight and obesity) factors that influence weight gain.

Diet. What you eat. What you *don't* eat. Both must be taken into account because you can eat a low-calorie diet and fail to lose fat, if your calories don't provide proper levels of protein, carbohydrates (fiber) and nutrition in the low-fat format needed for fat burn. The *source* of your calories has a greater effect on weight gain and weight loss than the *number* of your calories.

Exercise. (Including Daily Activity)The more sedentary you are, the greater your tendency for weight gain. The more fat you have to lose, the greater your need for exercise. You must burn more calories than you eat in order to lose fat, and there is a limit to the number of calories you can cut back. If you only cut calories, and do it indiscriminately, you can lose body muscle, which will in turn, cause you to burn less calories. Increasing your exercise and daily activity level is the only known way to burn enough calories while protecting your body muscle. This insures healthy weight loss and safeguards your weight maintenance.

Eating Patterns & Lifestyle. (Adult and Childhood)Your eating habits are learned behaviors that you gain over a lifetime and ingrain by repetition. Many eating problems carry over from your formative years and shape your lifestyle without your conscious awareness. Since poor eating habits re-inforce what you eat, why, how, when, and where you eat, they are weight-promoting, and can remain weight-promoting even after you've lost weight and think you are safe from fat. Changing these habits is the only known way to make your weight loss last.

Personality & Attitudes. Who you are and how you feel about yourself is both a reflection of weight, and an indicator of your potential success or failure. Low self-esteem and lack of assertiveness have been linked to excess weight. While no studies exist to identify specific personality profiles for *future* weight gainers, a wealth of data shows that self-strengthening is crucial to successful weight loss.

Aging. Your metabolic rate decreases with age, and this reduces your ability to burn calories as efficiently. While it is common for people to gain weight with age, it is not mandatory. With increased exercise and improved diet, you can remain slim in spite of the averages. You can raise your metabolic rate and lose weight at any age.

Genetics. This is the elusive territory you have no control over. It involves fat metabolism, fat cells, body heat and body type, along with a host of weight-gaining factors that may not be identified yet. For instance, many scientists are studying brown fat, thinking that may provide a link to why certain people gain weight and others lose it successfully. Others are studying genes and hormones and little trigger mechanisms in cells, looking for genetic causes of overweight and obesity. The wisest course is to leave genetics to researchers and concentrate on improving the factors that you can change, since they account for approximately 90% of the causes of overweight and obesity. A small minority of people (less than 1%) show genetic problems in relation to weight gain, and many can override their genetic tendencies with improvements in diet, exercise and behavior.

CELLULITE Lumpy fat, commonly found on hips, thighs and buttocks in women, and in the abdomen in men.

Fat leaves proportionately from your body, and unfortunately, you can't change fat. But you can change your diet and exercise patterns and that will take care of all of your fat, including the lumpy variety. But beware! Your diet has to protect your muscle (body protein) and be low-fat, and it must include the all food groups, otherwise you might wind up thinner, with lumpy bags. The combination of healthy diet and regular exercise builds your body muscle while it is removing fat. This gives you a firmer look all over at the end of your diet.

If you are over forty, or if you've had excess fat since childhood, it will take a little longer for the lumpy look to improve. Be patient and disciplined in your exercise. As your muscles strengthen and build up, the problem areas will become firmer. And don't forget, the places that have the most fat will be the last places to get thinner and firmer.

Cellulite and Liposuction

Forget about liposuction, unless you intend to stay on a very low fat diet after it. New fat will form in areas that didn't have fat before. Then you have lumpy fat somewhere else.

Cellulite Myths and Reality

There are two versions for the causes of cellulite — fad and fact. The Fad version is short and clever and the treatment list is long and expensive. The Fact version is complex and not selling anything, so the treatment is simple and inexpensive.

FAD DESCRIPTION	FACT DESCRIPTION
Cellulite is a special kind of fat created by waste products (toxins) and water trapped in fat cells and the tissues around fat cells.	All fat is the same. But fat distribution sites are different in men and women. Women tend to be lower body fat distributors, depositing more fat in hips, thighs and buttocks. Men tend to be upper body fat distributors, depositing more fat in abdomens and chests. Cell sizes differ. Hypertropic cells swell with fat and can increase to 5 times their size. Hyperplastic cells are smaller and more numerous — more cells store less fat over a greater cell area, giving a more level appearance. 1/2 your body fat is deposited directly under your skin, and women's outer layer of skin is thinner then men's. Therefore, women's fat, concentrated in the lower body in hypertrophic cells, can appear lumpier than men's fat in the same area.
FAD TREATMENTS	**FACT TREATMENT**
AT HOME: $10-40 each item loofas, special sponges, creams, cactus cloths, vitamin/mineral supplements, herbs, waffle-topped massagers, bath tonics, rubber suits, rollers, toners, electric muscle stimulators, spot reducing exercises. There's even a cream with hot pepper that makes skin red and tingly. **AT THE SPA:** $25-50 per treatment muscle stimulators, vibrating machines, whirlpools, air-streams, inflatable leggings, massages, thermal treatments, hormone injections, enzyme injections, wax treatments, heat.	Diet from the food groups, low fat Exercise to burn fat, and build muscle Drink water to flush out wastes

● **CELLULOSE** A type of fiber found in carbohydrate foods. Excellent weight loss food. *See* Fiber.

● **CEREALS** Grains. One of the required food groups. Grains are needed to round out your complete daily nutritional profile. But be cautious! Commercial cereals can be high sources of sugar and fat in the over-processed versions. Whole grain cereals are the preferred ones, especially with the bran and germ of the grain intact. They are the best nutrient and fiber sources, but check the labels to insure that they are low in fat and sugar. *See* Grains. Food Groups.

▲ **CHEWING** A factor in digestion. Also called Rate of Eating. Chewing your food slowly is an important aid to digestion, weight control, and hunger control. Carbohydrate digestion begins in your mouth with the help of enzymes from your salivary glands. When you eat too fast, and swallow too fast, carbohydrate digestion is limited in its first stage. What you eat is equally important, since processed carbohydrates have no fiber or texture, and lacking this consistency, chewing becomes minimal. Hunger takes approximately 20 minutes to abate from the time you begin eating, and chewing helps slow the eating process, so hunger ceases earlier in your meal. When you don't chew sufficiently and slow down the process, you can eat more calories without feeling satisfied, because hunger is still in full swing.

Eating faster doesn't mean speeding up your digestion, rather it's a form of bypassing the natural process of digestion. This can alter the whole cycle of digestion. Food arrives in your stomach in bulk and digestion is prolonged there. Enzymes in the stomach only break down protein. Carbohydrates that bypassed your mouth too quickly may have to wait to get broken down in your intestines along with fats. This prolongs digestion in your small intestines. All of these factors contribute to calories being stored. The result of a faster rate of eating is weight gain.

CHILDHOOD EATING PATTERNS Food and weight-related habits that were learned in childhood. These carry over to adulthood to form adult eating habits and lifestyle. They are part of the causes of overweight and obesity. *See* Habits. Causes.

● **CHOCOLATE** A derivative of the coffee bean. Chocolate contains the stimulants caffeine and theobromine, which speed up your central nervous system and heart beat. It also contains oxalic acid, which can interfere with your calcium absorption. So why do dieters love chocolate so much? Usually because of the added sugar and fat. Chocolate by itself is quite bitter, not a tempting food at all. If you have a real chocolate desire and want to lose weight, try carob instead. It's lower in fat, rich in B vitamins, minerals, and is similar in flavor to chocolate. It has no caffeine, and is non-allergenic.

You should limit your use of chocolate on a diet, but should you try to use willpower and deprivation to cut it out entirely? That will only send you straight to chocolate for a snack. A small mint patty can satisfy your chocolate desire with only 1 gram of fat. Cocoa can be substituted for a candy bar. The skillful dieter can still have chocolate and lose fat. If you believe the diets that say you can never have chocolate again, you're buying lack of trust in yourself, and an attitude that you have no control over food. When you believe that, you lose your control.

You can learn to make wise diet decisions that allow you variety and pleasure without adding fat. A decade of deprived dieting only proved it didn't work, because weight regain has become a major problem as a result. A good start is to get your baseline nutrition daily. That alone prevents a number of urges and desires that occur in a nutrient deficient state. With nutrition as your basis, you're healthier, you're in a better frame of mind to make good choices and stick to them. *See* Food Groups.

CHOLESTEROL A fatty substance produced in your liver and found in some foods.

Body Cholesterol. There are two kinds of cholesterol found in your body:

1. LDL. Low Density Lipoprotein. Called Bad Cholesterol. It carries cholesterol to your arteries where it can form deposits on the artery walls.
2. HDL. High Density Lipoprotein. Called Good Cholesterol. It picks up bad cholesterol and carries it back to your liver for excretion.

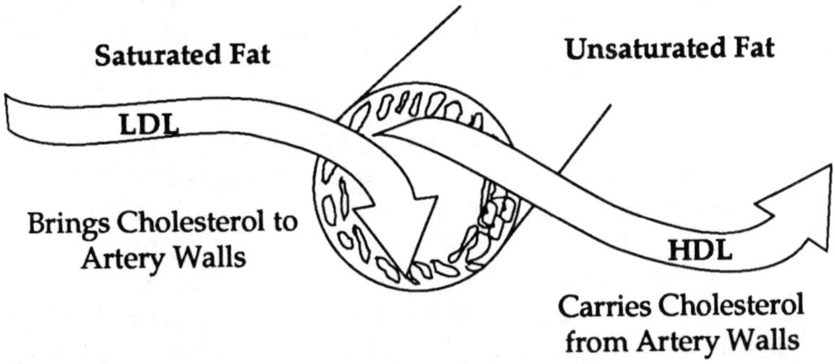

Lipoprotein literally means fat (lipid) plus protein. These fat/protein substances carry cholesterol through your bloodstream. When you have too much LDL, (carrying cholesterol), the excess can be deposited in your arteries and build up to form plaque. It is believed that the deposits occur in arteries that have been pre-damaged or stressed. The artery wall thickens with these deposits, and becomes less flexible, less capable of handling the blood flow. It's like water trying to pass through a clogged hose. The passage narrows from the deposits, the blood backs up, causing more pressure to push the blood through a smaller opening. Eventually an artery can completely close.

In an artery to the brain — this causes stroke. No blood to the brain.

In an artery to the heart — this causes heart attack. No blood to the heart.

In an artery elsewhere — this causes damage to tissues that require blood.

Food Cholesterol. Two types of food fat are associated with LDL and HDL — saturated fats and unsaturated fats.

1. Saturated Fats. Fats from animal sources, with the exception of coconut oil and palm oil. These fats are solid at room temperature, such as a stick of butter. If you equate this fat with your LDL, or bad cholesterol, it will make it easier to sort out fats. (This is the fat that leads to plaque deposits in arteries.)
2. Unsaturated Fats. Fats from vegetable sources. Corn oil, cottonseed oil, olive, soy. These fats are liquid at room temperature, such as bottled oils. If you equate this fat with your HDL, or good cholesterol, you'll know what you're looking for on labels. There are two kinds of unsaturated fats — Polyunsaturates, which actually raise the level of good cholesterol in your body, and Monounsaturates, which were thought to have no effect either way, but that opinion is beginning to change. The unsaturates, then, whether mono- or poly- are the best bets in fats.

SAT FATS — fats to limit UNSAT FATS — ok fats

Here's the tricky part. To get an UNSAT FAT oil to appear like butter and be useful as a spread, it has to be hardened. This is accomplished by a process called HYDROGENATION. The more hydrogenated a margarine is, the worse it is for you. The best choice of margarine, therefore, is the SOFTER one, because it is less hydrogenated. The softer margarines come in tubs. If you make the mistake of leaving one out on the counter, you'll see the oils separate. The stick margarines are more hydrogenated, and remain hard at room temperature.

Regardless of which type of margarine you buy, check the labels. After the total fat content, you'll see the numbers for SAT FAT AND UNSAT FAT. The first fat, and the most grams should be UNSATURATED. It might read UNSATURATED 5 AND SATURATED 2. That means you get 5 grams of unsaturated fat (OK fat) for every 2 grams of saturated fat (poor fat). That's considered a healthy ratio. If it's reversed, pass it by. If it says corn oil margarine, and the highest fat content says SATURATED OR HYDROGENATED, pass it by. Look for the lowest grams of SATURATED OR HYDROGENATED fat you can find on a margarine. If it doesn't tell you what kind of fat it contains, pass it by.

Because of this fat fandango, the best course would be to switch to apple butter and jams or jellies on your toast or muffin. They have no cholesterol. Cook exclusively with unsaturated oils. If you can't give up margarine on your toast or roll, at the least, switch to a tub margarine instead of a stick which is more hydrogenated. Many people came back to butter after evaluating the fat grams of both types of spreads, thinking butter was better tasting, and it contained the same number of total fat grams as margarine, so why not have the taste? Cholesterol is why not. The more you can limit the cholesterol, the less risk you'll have of plaque buildup on your artery walls.

➡ How To Lower Your Cholesterol

Many people who have tried to lower their cholesterol have been disappointed in the results. Cutting fat isn't enough. Increasing your fiber has been shown to have a more dramatic effect on cholesterol levels. Also studies on lecithin show that it has the interesting ability to hold cholesterol in solution, so it doesn't deposit.

You can get lecithin from soy products, which are excellent protein foods. Also niacin has been found to help reduce cholesterol, and you can find that in poultry and grains. If you add exercise as a booster, you'll see your cholesterol level come down, since exercise raises the level of HDL (good cholesterol).

The guidelines for cholesterol reduction are:

Reduce total fat intake
Reduce saturated fat intake
Increase unsaturated fat intake
Eat less cholesterol in your diet
Eat more complex carbohydrates (for fiber, lecithin, niacin)
Exercise
If you smoke, stop

The above list sounds complicated to someone who doesn't study fat for an occupation, but you can turn to *cholesterol at a glance,* which combines all of these factors into a quick view of where your cholesterol is coming from, and how to get the better variety of fats.

Cholesterol Tests. Your cholesterol level can change at different times. In fact, you can have it done twice in the same day at different places and get different readings, depending on how accurate the measurement was. Naturally, you'd like to go home with the lower number in mind and have a double cheese pizza with cholesterol in the cheese. But for your health's sake, you should get regular tests at your physician's office, to get your cholesterol RANGE. If your cholesterol remains high, that's cause for concern. In the meantime, you can make the adjustments in your diet and exercise, and you will be accomplishing what the doctor will tell you to do. Some people need medication, so it's best to check your level at every annual physical.

When you have your body cholesterol checked, it is a reading of both your good cholesterol (HDL) and bad cholesterol (LDL). You can have a borderline LDL level, and a high HDL level, and it is not as risky as a high LDL level and low HDL level. The key is in the ratio between the cholesterols.

The recommended level is:

LDL Level: less than 130 mg/dl. (DL means deciliter of blood.)
HDL Level: more than 35 mg/dl.

The total cholesterol level ratings are:

Desirable	199 mg/dl or lower
Borderline	200-239 mg/dl
Too high	240 mg/dl or higher

Cholesterol Medications. Even when you have a high cholesterol level, the first course of action is to try diet and exercise improvements. If that fails, medications are recommended. However, these medications still require that you change your diet and exercise, so it's best to do it the first time. Recent evidence shows that the medications combined with diet and exercise actually remove the plaque buildup. If plaque buildup continues unabated, balloon surgery — angeoplasty, or heart surgery may be required.

The medications for cholesterol reduction are called antihyperlipidemics, meaning they reduce the excess lipid concentration. The most commonly used medications are:

1. Clofibrate. This medication is not considered as safe as others because of increased deaths from non-coronary causes (36% higher).
2. Cholestramine. Colestipol. These work in the stomach, and are therefore considered safer. They can cause constipation, nausea, vomiting, flatulence, and

diarrhea, but the symptoms often abate as use continues.

3. Niacin. This can create gastric distress, and more frequent cardiac arrhythmias, and possible liver dysfunction.
4. Neomycin. Probucol. These can cause mild diarrhea. Often a combination of these medications are used.
5. MEVACOR. A newer medication that selectively lowers LDL cholesterol.

How To Avoid Cholesterol Confusion

Best Sources of Food: low cholesterol foods, with little saturated fat.— vegetables, grains, fruits. Eat Hearty!

Cholesterol and saturated fats are justified in lean meats and poultry, because the other nutrients ARE ESSENTIAL. Don't get afraid of meats because of their cholesterol content. When you eliminate the main sources— eggs, butter, fatty dairy products, and cheese, lean meats are moderate sources of cholesterol, and the saturated fat content is not way out of proportion to the unsaturated fat. Enjoy!

Least Best: Cholesterol content is high for the portion size, despite nutrient composition. Most cheeses, butter, lard, creams, ice cream, and desserts that contain these ingredients are high cholesterol. When you eliminate two or three of your main sources, you'd be surprised how much you take out of your diet.

Easiest Solution: Avoid or limit the highest cholesterol foods and switch to vegetable oils for cooking. Get fiber in your diet, and exercise. Check the next two lists for the highest sources of cholesterol in regular food and desserts.

Recommended maximum of cholesterol is *300* mg/day.

12 CHOLESTEROL ELEVATORS

EGG YOLK (1)	312 mg
*8 CLAMS	240 mg
*4 OZ LOBSTER	225 mg
4 OZ BACON	249 mg
4 OZ LIVER (CKN)	629 mg
*4 OZ CRAB	113 mg
1 HOT DOG	74 mg
4 OZ DARK TURKEY	114 mg
1 CUP SOUR CREAM	102 mg
4 PATS OF BUTTER	140 mg
1 CUP RICOTTA	124 mg
2 SLICES MOST CHEESE	54 mg

A BACON DOUBLE CHEESEBURGER WILL TOP YOUR DAILY CHOLESTEROL MAXIMUM.

8 TOP CHOLESTEROL DESSERTS

1 PIECE OF CHEESECAKE	163 mg
1 PIECE OF APPLE PIE	156 mg
1 PIECE OF SPONGE CAKE	123 mg
1 PIECE LEMON MERINGUE PIE	130 mg
1 SERVING BREAD PUDDING	170 mg
1 ECLAIR	145 mg
1 PIECE OF CUSTARD PIE	278 mg
1 PIECE OF PUMPKIN PIE	91 mg

REMEMBER THAT SWEETS OR PASTRIES WITH CHEESE, CUSTARD, EGGS, CREAM OR BUTTER WILL NATURALLY BE HIGH CHOLESTEROL.

For the exact count of cholesterol, sat and unsat, see the EZ Cholesterol Counter on the following pages.

*Fish are being reevaluated in terms of cholesterol, because of omega 3 oils. However, these are still high fat compared to other fish, and two of them are often dipped in butter for eating.

ez cholesterol counter

The primary sources of cholesterol are high-fat dairy products, high-fat meats, and processed desserts with added fats. When you moderate these sources of cholesterol, it really makes a difference.

The complex carbohydrates are cholesterol-beaters, since they are high in fiber and low in unsaturated fat. You don't need to count them, just increase them to reduce your LDL and raise your HDL.

EZ CHOLESTEROL COUNTER.

Dairy 1 cup

	TFAT	CHO	SAT	UNSAT
Buttermilk	2	9	1	.7
Chocolate Milk	8	30	5	3
Condensed	27	114	17	8
Dried Whole	34	124	21	11
Dried Whole Instant	65	1190	0	29
Dried Nonfat	.9	24	.6	T
Evaporated Whole	19	74	12	7
Evaporated Skim	.5	10	.3	.2
Goat	10	28	7	3
Human	1	4	06	06
Low Fat Milk	5	18	3	2
Malted Milk	10	37	6	3
Skim Milk	T	4	T	T
Whole Milk	8	33	5	3
Creams 1 cup				
Half & Half	28	89	17	9
Heavy Cream	88	326	55	29
Sour Cream	49	102	30	16
Milk Deserts 1 cup				
Ice Cream	14	59	9	5
Iced Milk	6	18	4	2
Sherbert	4	14	2	1
Yogurt	7	29	5	2
Yogurt Low Fat	3	14	2	1
Yogurt Low Fat, Fruit	3	12	2	1
Eggs 1				
Egg Large	5	312*	2	2
Egg Small	4	219	1	2
Egg Whites	0	0	0	0
Eggnog	19	149	11	7

*One large egg is more cholesterol than the recommended daily maximum

Oils and Fats 1 Teaspoon

	TFAT	CHO	SAT	UNSAT
Bacon Fat	14	—	6	4
Butter	12	35	101	66
Chicken Fat	14	—	—	—
Lard	13	12	5	7
Margarine Stick	14	0	2	9*
Margarine Tub	7	0	1	6*
Cod Liver Oil	14	119	0	0
Corn Oil	14	T	1	11
Cottonseed	14	0	3	9
Olive	14	T	1	11
Peanut	14	T	2	10
Safflower	14	T	1	12
Soybean	14	T	2	10
Sesame	14	T	2	11
Sunflower	14	T	2	12
Wheat Germ Oil	14	T	2	9
Vegetable Shortening	12	—	3	9

*Margarines differ in saturated and unsaturated content. The best choice is tub margarine, because it requires less hydrogenation (is softer at room temperature). However, even tub levels can differ. Check the label to be sure.

Cheeses 1 Ounce or 1 Slice

	TFAT	CHO	SAT	UNSAT
American Cheddar	9	27	6	3
Blue	8	21	5	2
Brick	8	27	5	3
Brie	8	28	0	0
Camembert	7	20	4	2
Cheddar	9	30	6	3
Cheese Spread	6	16	4	2
Colby	9	27	6	3
Cream Cheese	11	31	6	4
Edam	8	25	5	2
Gouda	8	32	5	2

	TFAT	CHO	SAT	UNSAT
Gruyere	9	31	5	3
Limburger	8	26	5	3
Monterey	9	—	—	—
Mozzarella	6	22	4	2
Mozzarella Skim	5	15	3	2
Muenster	9	27	5	3
Parmesan Hard	7	19	5	2
Parmesan Grated	1	4	1.5 (1 Tbsp)	
Port duSalut	8	35	5	3
Provolone	8	20	5	2
Roquefort	9	26	5	3
Swiss	8	26	5	2
Swiss Pasteurized	7	24	5	2
Softer Cheeses 1 cup				
Cottage Cheese	9	31	6	3
2% Cottage Cheese	4	19	3	1
Ricotta	32	124	20	10
Ricotta Skim	19	9	12	6
Cheese Souffle	16	159	9	7

Desserts, Sweets

	TFAT	CHO	SAT	UNSAT
Brownies	9	25	1	6
1 piece of Sponge Cake	2	123	1	1
Custard	14	278	7	6
Apple Pie	17	156	5	12
Lemon Meringue	14	130	4	8
Pumpkin Pie	16	91	5	9
Pudding (Bread)	16	170	8	5
Cheesecake	26	163	6	6
Eclair	13	145	4	6

Meats, Poultry 4 oz.

These are listed in 4 ounce serving sizes, since that's the most common serving that people eat. But note that the recommended daily allowance is 2 ounces.

	TFAT	CHO	SAT	UNSAT
Bacon	80	249	25	45
Beef				
Chuck Roast	19	67	9	8
Ground,Lean	11	74	5	5
Ground,Reg	24	77	12	11
Rib Roast	39	65	18	18
Rump Roast	24	65	19	19
Bologna	33	208	13	17
Braunschweiger	31	—	11	16
Canadian Bacon	16	100	6	8
Chicken				
Back	10	92	3	6
Breast	4	60	1	3
Drumstick	7	60	2	4
Liver	5	629	2	2
Neck	5	92	0	0
Thigh	8	92	2	5
Wing	13	92	4	8
Chili w/beans	15	0	7	7
Club Steak	33	65	16	15
Duck	32	80	8	20
Flank Steak	6	65	3	3
Frankfurters	32	74	12	18
Goose	38	—	10	22
Ham Cured	34	80	12	17
Knockwurst	36	84	14	17
Lamb				
Leg	15	66	8	6
Chops	24	68	13	9
Shoulder	23	68	13	9
Pheasant	13	—	4	7
Polish Sausage	29	0	10	16

	TFAT	CHO	SAT	UNSAT
Pork				
Chops	22	65	8	11
Pork Link Sausage	57	0	20	29
Rabbit	7	73	3	3
Sausage,				
Blood	41	0	0	0
Country Style	35	0	12	18
Salami	38	0	13	22
Vienna (7)	22	0	0	0
Steaks				
Flank Steak	6	65	3	3
Porterhouse Steak	37	65	18	17
Round Steak	13	65	6	6
Sirloin Steak	28	65	13	12
T-Bone Steak	42	65	17	22
Turkey				
Dark	9	114	2	6
Light	4	87	1	2
Canned	6	0	2	4
Veal				
Breast	15	63	7	7
Chuck	9	80	4	4
Cutlet	10	63	5	4
Rib Roast	12	63	6	5
Rump	8	63	3	3
Venison	4	0	3	4

Fish

	TFAT	CHO	SAT	UNSAT
Abalone	T	—	0	0
Anchovy	T	5	0	0
Bass	2	—	T	T
Bluefish	3	—	0	0
Carp	5	—	T	3
Catfish	3	—	1	2
Caviar (1 tsp)	T	7	—	—
Clams (4)	2	120	—	—

	TFAT	CHO	SAT	UNSAT
Clams Canned	T	240	—	—
Cod	T	57	T	T
Crab, Steamed	2	113	—	—
Crab, Canned	4	161	—	—
Eel	21	57	5	7
Flounder	1	57	T	T
Frogs Legs	T	10	—	—
Haddock	7	68	T	T
Halibut	1	56	T	T
Herring	7	96	2	4
Lobster	2	225	—	—
Mackerel	11	107	3	7
Oysters	2	56	—	—
Oysters, Canned	1	27	T	T
Perch Ocean	2	—	T	T
Perch, Yellow	1	80	—	—
Pike	1	—	T	T
Pollock	1	—	T	T
Salmon, Fresh	15	68	T	T
Salmon, Canned	3	19	1	T
Sardines oil, drained	12	80	—	—
Scallops	T	39	—	—
Shad	11	—	—	—
Shrimp, Fresh		172	—	—
Shrimp, Canned	T	48	—	—
Smelt	2	—	—	—
Snails	T	—	—	—
Snapper	1	—	T	T
Swordfish	4	—	—	—
Trout	12	62	2	3
Tuna, Oil (drained)	13	104	5	6
Tuna, Water	1	126	—	—
Whitefish	9	—	T	4

(—) Not Available

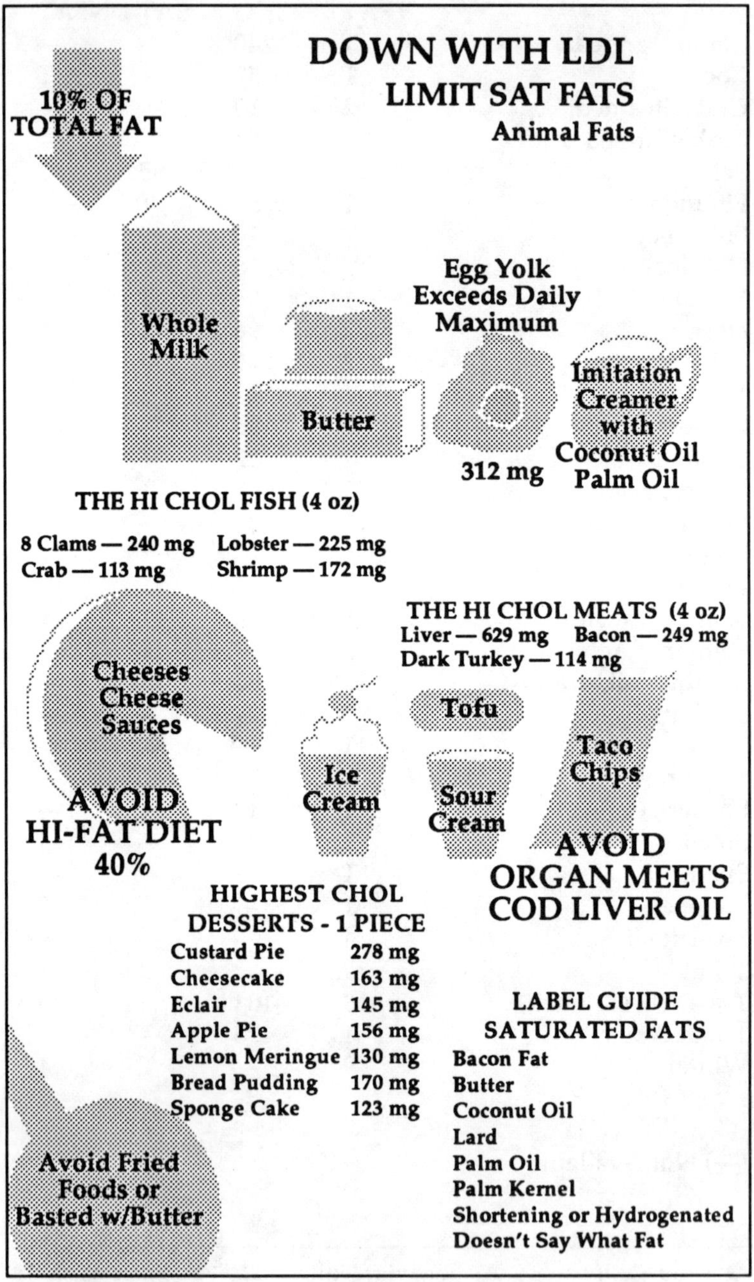
DOWN WITH LDL
LIMIT SAT FATS
Animal Fats
10% OF
TOTAL FAT
Whole
Milk
Butter
Egg Yolk
Exceeds Daily
Maximum
312 mg
Imitation
Creamer
with
Coconut Oil
Palm Oil
THE HI CHOL FISH (4 oz)
8 Clams — 240 mg
Lobster — 225 mg
Crab — 113 mg
Shrimp — 172 mg
THE HI CHOL MEATS (4 oz)
Liver — 629 mg
Bacon — 249 mg
Dark Turkey — 114 mg
Cheeses
Cheese
Sauces
Tofu
Taco
Chips
Ice
Cream
Sour
Cream
AVOID
HI-FAT DIET
40%
AVOID
ORGAN MEETS
COD LIVER OIL
HIGHEST CHOL
DESSERTS - 1 PIECE
Custard Pie 278 mg
Cheesecake 163 mg
Eclair 145 mg
Apple Pie 156 mg
Lemon Meringue 130 mg
Bread Pudding 170 mg
Sponge Cake 123 mg
LABEL GUIDE
SATURATED FATS
Bacon Fat
Butter
Coconut Oil
Lard
Palm Oil
Palm Kernel
Shortening or Hydrogenated
Doesn't Say What Fat
Avoid Fried
Foods or
Basted w/Butter

UP WITH HDL

INCREASE UNSAT FAT

Vegetable Fats

10% OF TOTAL FAT

Low-Fat or Skim Milk

Any Vegetable Oil (Not Hydrogenated)

Best Choice Tub Margarine

Egg Whites

Margarine Corn Oil Or Other Polyunsat

EAT LEAN MEATS
POULTRY WITHOUT SKIN

❤ **SPECIAL EFFECTS:**
Lecithin from Soy*
Niacin from Poultry
Fiber from Apple

•Restaurant•
Say: "Cook without butter no cheese sauce."

LOW FAT DIET 25%

EAT MORE COMPLEX CARBOHYDRATES

Veg
Fruits
Grains

EXERCISE!
AEROBIC 3X WEEK
30 Minutes (Raises HDL)

LABEL GUIDE
UNSATURATED FATS
Corn Oil
Cottonseed
Olive
Peanut
Sunflower
Soy Bean
Sesame
Wheat Germ
Vegetable
Look for least "Hydrogenated"

Cook Stir Fry with Polyunsat
Broil
Bake Butter Free

*Keeps LDL in suspension. Prevents deposits.

CIRCULATION Blood movement through arteries and veins to deliver oxygen to tissues and take away waste products and carbon dioxide. Your rate of circulation has an indirect effect on weight gain, but the effect can be significant. Blood circulation facilitates many processes that are central to fat burn. It carries oxygen to your muscles, where fat burn occurs; it carries nutrients from your intestines to your cells for metabolism; it carries vitamins and minerals to your cells, which are essential for the chemical reactions of metabolism; it carries wastes away from your cells after metabolism; it carries salt to your kidneys which aid in their elimination. All of these processes are part of your internal calorie regulating cycle that better circulation can enhance. You can improve your circulation with regular exercise and diaphragm breathing, earning double benefits. The exercise burns calories and breathing exercises help you stay calm when stressed.

● **COLAS** Drinks with 100% sugar. *See* Sugar.

▲ **COMMITMENT** The deal you make with yourself. The amount of energy, time and effort you make to make your diet succeed. The trust you place in yourself. The pledge you keep.

Commitment is a very critical factor in successful dieting. It's important to understand that you're not making a commitment to a particular diet plan, a contract to a clinic, or a pledge to your favorite counselor or nurse who weighs you, even though these people are there to help you keep your commitment. The only pledge that works is the one you make to yourself. That way, if there's a snowstorm one day and the roads are closed, you won't stop dieting because you can't check in to get weighed.

To help you make the best pledge you can make to yourself, try not to jump into a diet on impulse – because a wedding or reunion is coming up – unless you plan to go the distance to ideal body weight. The more you start and stop diets, the harder it will be to believe the commitment you make to yourself. Choose a diet carefully, and don't buy into it if you have any doubts about your ability to comply with it. Ask questions, and if you are unsatisfied with the answers, find another program. Try to find a diet that doesn't feel like punishment, and there are many around. Avoid gimmicks and extra purchases if you can, since real fresh food is the best fuel for energy and fat burn. Don't hesitate to call other people who have been on the diet and ask their opinions. Use every resource at your disposal to make your decision, and take your time making it. It's better to wait and make your commitment real, than to start too quickly, without being ready to make the changes you will need in your lifestyle. Once you make your decision, stick to it! You'll prove to yourself that you can succeed at other things.

▲ **COMPLIANCE** Adhering to a diet program, following the rules and regulations.

Many dieters have problems with compliance for a variety of reasons.

1. The diet you choose doesn't fit into your lifestyle. The plan you use for weight loss should be one that is comfortable to do, or you won't continue doing it for long. When a diet causes too much disruption of your normal routines, it becomes stressful and a chore, and you find yourself getting angry at a hundred little things. Eventually, these emotions lead to a break from the plan. Diets that are too far out of line with everyday life aren't much use to you over the long term, they can create new problems instead of resolving your old ones. One of the reasons dieters choose unfitting plans is because they see a diet as a form of short-term punishment that has to be endured for the purpose of weight loss. This doesn't have to be you, if you close the gap in your mind between "diet" and everyday life, and select a program that makes

you feel positive about working toward health on a daily basis.

2. The diet you choose is too regimented and repetitive. A diet doesn't have to be a robot-like routine where you do everything someone else tells you to do, blindly following rules, feeling that if you don't you'll gain weight. On diets like this, when you find yourself breaking the rules, you don't tell anyone, because you feel guilty, like a kid with your hand in the cookie jar. While diets involve discipline, weight loss is not an either/or situation. Their way or no way. The one and only solution. Before entering a program, ask to see the menus and rules. Be sure you have a clear picture of what's in store for you, so you won't be disappointed later. Don't sign on to a program because the girl at the front desk is fun to talk to. Sign on because it offers what you want and shows you what your getting. If they tell you that their rules and food lists are private information that can only be divulged to a client, go someplace where weight loss isn't treated like a big secret.
3. You are half-hearted about dieting. This can be because you see dieting as an unpleasant experience, when it doesn't have to be. Or you can be afraid to go through the process and face another failure. Or you may have convinced yourself that you were born to be fat. There are as many reasons for this as there are dieters. Make sure you're ready to make a change in your eating habits and lifestyle, before you take on the project. If you're not quite ready, don't make the investment. Losing and gaining can be worse for you in the long run. Explore the reasons you might feel reluctant to diet, and make an effort to resolve these conflicts before you start dieting. Give yourself time to get ready to make a real commitment. That way you'll be setting yourself up for success.
4. You jumped into the plan too quickly. Don't buy into a diet because a wedding is coming up in two weeks. Do

it because you want to lose your excess weight for life. Don't let the immediate stress of weight cause you to sign with the first program you find. The faster you jump in, the faster you will jump out. Each time you do that, you lose a little belief that you can work out your weight problems. If a wedding is coming up in two weeks and you want to lose weight, go for a brisk walk and think about the marriage of low-fat eating and regular exercise and what it can do for you. Then just start doing it.

5. You want instant results. This is the biggest reason people quit diets. False expectations. Rapid weight loss. It's also the reason people regain weight so fast. The faster you lose, the faster you regain. You didn't gain your excess weight overnight, and you're only hurting yourself if you plan to lose it within a week or two. If this was the only change you made in your weight loss perspective, it would be the best one you could do. When you want instant results, you choose plans that promise instant results, and you get what you ask for. So ask for something else. Ask for lasting weight loss and enjoy seeing the slow, steady changes in your weight and wellbeing on a weekly basis. They're the ones that comply with a lean life.

▲ **CONFIDENCE** The surety that you will succeed with your goals, based on support skills (not willpower). *See* Control.

CONSTIPATION Intestinal slowdown. This can be caused by a variety of factors:

You're not drinking enough water.

You're not eating enough fiber, OR you increased your fiber intake too fast, and didn't drink water simultaneously. If you drink water when you increase your fiber, you will not have problems with fiber. Fiber binds with water in your intestines and speeds up your food transit time. But it's got to have water to do it.

You're not chewing sufficiently, swallowing too fast, and eating too rapidly. This throws off the natural process of digestion at the outset.

You're too stressed or anxious while eating. This can tighten your diaphragm and stomach muscles and interfere with digestion. Before you eat, five minutes of deep breathing will let go of the stress and tension.

You're eating too late at night, particularly heavy proteins. Late night eating doesn't give your food time to digest. Your metabolism slows down dramatically when you sleep, and you aren't digesting the food properly.

Your diet is imbalanced on a regular basis. This makes everything work less efficiently.

You're not getting enough exercise. Exercise increases your food transit time and keeps food from lingering in your intestines where it can stagnate.

Constipation may also be other medical conditions. If it is severe or prolonged, see your doctor.

▲ **CONTINGENCY PLAN** A coping skill to use for emergency situations. A problem-solving technique. During weight loss, contingency plans center around food and eating problems, such as meal-pre-planning, developing strategies for eating out at parties, restaurants, vacations, and planning behavior substitutes like exercise, breathing exercise and relaxation to replace your usual emergency eating habits.

In maintenance, your contingency plans are more geared to relapse prevention, or weight regain. This means taking action *before* you regain 10 pounds, so you don't have to get caught in the cycle of losing and regaining excessive amounts of weight. Most dieters never take the time to develop successful coping skills and contingency plans during their diet routine. They see *weight loss* as their only diet goal, and even if they achieve it, they are stranded at ideal weight without the skills to keep it. Gradually, they fall back into old habits, because they have not developed controls to prevent this. Coping skills act as *controls* – habits you can use on a regular basis for fitness insurance. Without these skills, weight loss is seldom permanent. *See* ▲ topics for coping skills, especially Lifestyle.

▲ **CONTROL** Taking charge of, or authority over. To direct.

Anyone who has ever been on a diet has heard the word control. It's the byword of most commercial programs. Control your appetite. Control your portions. Control your will. Control yourself.

Weight gain is seen as loss of control, and weight loss is seen as taking control.

The problem is, control is like the two-headed monster. When you start to take control, you feel great and in control. Then the other face turns and you feel the overwhelming tension of having to be in control all the time. Control starts to control you, and you feel like you're going to break. The easiest way to get out of control, is to think you can control everything in your life at the same time.

Control isn't what you really need on a diet. What you really need is to OWN your decisions, actions, habits and lifestyle. You need to feel part of it, in charge — but flexible, able to *go with the flow* without losing your sense of self support. That's very different from control.

Take stress, as an example. If you tell someone to take control over stress, it can make them feel more stressed. First, it assumes they have no control, and are deficient. Working from a feeling of deficiency isn't a positive headset, directed to positive goals. Secondly, it puts the blame on the person, who seemingly lost control. Working from a feeling of blame and guilt isn't self-supporting or productive. Third, it's a paradox. More people get stressed from needing too much control and not getting it, than people who let go of the need for control, and rely on step-by-step decisions about health.

Willpower is an example of a control technique.

You're supposed to exercise your "no"-power over foods you think you want. The more you try to resist the food, the greater the hold of that food. You think about it all the time. You visit the food in supermarkets and stare at it, saying no. You dream about it at night. Finally, one day, when no one's looking (not even you), you go out and get that food. You eat it until you satisfy the three-week obsession you had, while saying no.

Skillpower is an OWNING technique. You own your desire for that food. What are you going to do about it? Know the food inside out, what it does and doesn't provide in nutrition and fat-burn. Study your reactions and desires for the food. How does it get to you, when and why? How does it make you feel after you eat it? Guilty? Temporarily satisfied? Happy? Admit what you really feel and deal with it. Make reasonable choices. Gradually limit your dependence on that food, by replacing it with healthier alternatives. If you're going to faint without a slice of cake, have a sliver, then go back to limiting it in your life. When something owns you, no matter how small (a truffle), it is something worth dealing with. It won't go away by itself. You own it, you have to let it go.

As adults, most of us have a number of different factors in our lives that we control, and do reasonably well at it. To buy the idea that you are out of control because you are overweight, is neither helpful nor particularly accurate. Thin people can be out of control in areas of their life that you are skilled at handling. The best way to view your weight and food problems are *as an issue* you want to deal with. List the issue as a priority, and think about the choices you can make and want to make. Step by step, change one unhealthy food habit into a healthy one. One day, you'll turn around and find that your efforts have dominoed, since one healthy habit leads to another and another. One day, you'll own your new habits and health. *See* Eating Habits.

● **COOKING** How you treat what you eat. To create a healthy, low-fat lifestyle, you need to set up a kitchen that will promote easy cooking, while you give yourself a whole new view of eating and cooking without fats, sugars and sodium. This means that you don't want a kitchen that looks deprived or depressed, stripped of food and pleasure. You want a kitchen that is ALIVE with pleasure and energy, so that cooking low-fat becomes a gourmet delight.

Try to enjoy the pleasure of cooking while you are on a diet. If you only rely on microwave dinners or oven entrees in a box, you deny yourself the smell of food, and the sensual pleasure that comes from preparing a good meal, with hot and cold fares.

How To Design Your Diet Kitchen

1. Start by adding a spice rack full of herbs and spices, free of the ingredients that give you too much sodium. You might even consider taking pottery as a hobby (to substitute for eating), and you can make your own herb and spice jars. Make your herb and spice rack a real eye catcher with fresh cinnamon sticks, and perhaps a planter of fresh basil, so the sight and smell can permeate your kitchen, giving you a new feeling about cooking with low-fat pleasure. Use herbs and spices for flavoring in sauces and sautes. Lemon, garlic and basil are excellent for fish. Orange, basil and whole wheat flour make a delicious, cream-like sauce for chicken. Use your imagination to create your own herb and spice combinations to replace the butter you may have used in the past.
2. Set up a rack of unsaturated oils to use instead of butter or margarine. There are many, including peanut oil, cottonseed oil, olive oil. You can find a collection of bottles that will show off the oils, and you might think of painting designs on the bottles yourself. If you keep a rack of the varieties of unsaturated oils that are available, you won't feel so

limited when you're cooking low fat. Different oils have subtle taste differences, and you can experiment with herbs and spice mixes to make your own oil mixes. Keep a selection of wine vinegars on your rack of oils. There are many varieties and the colors will be pleasing to your eye.

◆ **COOL DOWNS** A mild exercise or stretch for a minimum of five minutes after a vigorous exercise. This prevents that after-exercise ache or soreness in your muscles by breaking down lactic acid which can build up if oxygen supply to your muscles is limited (as in anaerobic exercise). In addition, it allows you to bring your heart rate down gradually, instead of abruptly. The cooling effect occurs as your body heat is reduced and your temperature returns to normal. You can use a brief easy walk for a cool down exercise, or repeat the full body stretch or yoga you used as a warm up. *See* Warm Ups. Stretches.

◆ **CROSS COUNTRY SKIING** Skill sport aerobic exercise. *See* Exercise.

◆ **CROSS TRAINING** A combination of exercises that include endurance, strength, flexibility, and aerobic conditioning.A method for exercise versatility, and best effect. An example of cross training might be: On Monday, you power walk. On Tuesday, you do Stretching Exercises. On Wednesday, you Walk, and so on through the week. The next week you might want to develop more upper body strength, so on Monday, you weight lift, on Tuesday you Stretch, on Wednesday you Power Walk, on Thursday, you Stretch, The goal is to combine weight bearing exercises, with flexibility exercises to gain strength along with grace. It also combats boredom with exercise for high achievers.

d

◆ **DAILY ACTIVITY** Routine motion that produces heat and burns calories. The more active you are on a daily basis, the greater your metabolic rate. Activity levels can be responsible for burning 25% of your calories. It doesn't take a great deal of effort to activate your daily life. If you have a desk job, get up and move around on breaks. Walk to the store sometimes, instead of taking your car. Use more stairs than elevators, and park farther away from your destination. Use the seasonal opportunities to get outside, rake leaves, shovel snow, landscape around the house. If you live in an apartment, you might find a trampoline easy for exercise, since there's no impact on the floor. You can walk on it, run, or bounce. Take up an outdoor sport, preferably not one that lets you stand around a great deal, like golf. The little activities add up, even though you might think they don't mean much. They help you become a more active person overall, then it's easier to think about starting an aerobic program for real fat burn. *See* Exercise.

● **DAIRY PRODUCTS** One of the daily essential food groups. Animal sources of protein, calcium, riboflavin, vitamins and minerals. The recommended servings daily are: 2 Servings for an Adult, 4 Servings for Teens, 3 Servings for Children, 4 Servings for Pregnant and

Lactating Women. The best source is the low-fat version. Dieters often forego their calcium, thinking that milk and milk products are fattening. This is a harmful habit, since lack of calcium can lead to osteoporosis — dry and brittle bones, and it can upset your protein balance, leading to muscle losses. Less muscle means more fat gain. *See* Calcium. Food Groups.

◆ **DANCING** A daily activity exercise, non-aerobic (unless it's break dancing for 30 minutes sustained). *See* Exercise.

◆ **DANCE AEROBICS** Aerobic exercise to music.

Benefits:

- Full-body workout.
- Easily accessible — from health spas and community centers to home use with video and audio tapes and instructional guides.
- Entertaining, incorporating high-energy music.

Guidelines:

- Check the credentials of the instructor; he or she should have formal training or certification in physical fitness rather than just "liking to dance."
- Assess the facility: type of floor surface (wood preferred); amount of ventilation; average number in class.
- Find out about the levels of classes offered: how they differ in length of class, degree of difficulty and supervision, length of warmup and cool-down periods, frequency of supervised heart rate monitoring.
- Join the best program that offers low-to high-level classes and take responsibility for yourself. Use target heart rate to avoid overexertion; forcing yourself to "keep up" is more harmful than not dancing at all.
- Always warm up. Never just jump into a class late. If

you arrive late, take time to do your own warm up first.

- Wear good, supportive shoes. *See* Exercise.

DEFICIENCY Lack of one or more essential nutrients needed for body growth, repair and maintenance. Nutrient deficiencies can occur for a variety of reasons.

1. Improper eating. You can overeat and be deficient in your daily nutrients if you are not eating a balanced diet from the daily food groups. Or you can be eating certain energy to excess, such as sugar, which will deplete other nutrient sources. Taking one vitamin to excess will throw off the others. Excess protein can deplete calcium from your bones. That's why it's so vital to be sure you get balanced nutrition, regardless of the amount of food you eat. Your metabolism requires all of the daily nutrients in the food groups to function properly, and that also means burning fat better as well.
2. Metabolic Disorder. You can have deficiencies if you have an inability to digest or metabolize certain nutrients, as in diabetes, where carbohydrates cannot be metabolized, or you can have a problem with lactose metabolism, which can cause nutrient deficiencies to occur.
3. Prolonged Stress. The stress response speeds up your body processes, including your heart rate and metabolism. This causes your nutrients to be burned off faster, and can result in deficiencies.
4. Illnesses, injuries or surgery can cause nutrient deficiencies, since the body needs more energy for repair.
5. Weight loss diets are a common source of nutrient deficiency, since many dieters feel that anything is acceptable if it gets rid of fat. But beware! Nutrient deficient diets don't get rid of much fat at all. They get rid of your body muscle and water, and that adds

more fat.

6. Obesity. You can have major nutrient deficiencies if you have obesity. Your fat mass steals your nutrition, and keeps your nutrients out of balance on a regular basis. That's why obesity is considered a disease of *malnutrition,* instead of a disease caused by overeating. You can eat the same calories as a normal-weight person, but gain weight, because nutritional deficiencies keep you in a fat-gaining cycle. *See* Food Groups, for nutrient needs.

DEHYDRATION An excessive loss of body fluids and water. This condition should not be confused with *mild* fluid loss, and needs medical attention if the condition persists. However, dehydration can occur if you exercise in a hot, dry climate without taking water breaks to replace lost fluids. Or it can occur on severely imbalanced diets,which allow water losses. The immediate solution is to drink plenty of water on a steady, regular basis, not all in one gulp. Also cut back on your salt intake. If the condition does not improve in a day or two, see your doctor.

DESIRABLE BODY WEIGHT The best weight you can be for your height, frame size and sex. *See* Ideal Weight for height/weight tables.

DIABETES/MELLITUS A disease of the pancreas. Known as *sweet urine* because of the increased concentration of sugar excreted in the urine.

There are two types of diabetes.

TYPE I Insulin Dependent. The pancreas produces no insulin, or low insulin. This results in an inability to metabolize carbohydrates, since insulin is needed to convert glucose to energy for metabolism. The unmetabolized glucose remains in the blood and accumulates. This can lead to coma or death. 10% of all diabetes is the insulin-dependent type, requiring insulin injections.

TYPE II Non-insulin Dependent. The pancreas produces insulin, but excess fat prevents the body from using insulin, creating an *insulin resistance.* As a result, the pancreas has to make larger amounts of insulin to metabolize carbohydrates. 90% of all diabetes is the insulin-resistant type. It can be brought on by excessive intake of sugar, and obesity. This type can be treated by weight loss and proper nutrition.

UPPER BODY FAT DISTRIBUTORS HAVE A GREATER RISK OF DEVELOPING DIABETES.

PEOPLE WHO ARE OBESE HAVE 3 TIMES THE RISK OF DIABETES, WHILE PEOPLE WHO HAVE UPPER BODY FAT AND OBESITY, HAVE 10 TIMES THE RISK.

SINCE MEN ARE PRIMARILY UPPER BODY FAT DISTRIBUTORS, OBESITY IN MEN PRESENTS A GREATER RISK OF DIABETES.

SYMPTOMS OF DIABETES INCLUDE LOSS OF WEIGHT, INCREASED APPETITE, EXCESSIVE THIRST, FREQUENT URINATION, VISION PROBLEMS, SKIN ITCHES, POOR HEALING. IT MUST BE TREATED BY A PHYSICIAN.

● **DIARY, FOOD** A daybook of eating habits. The story of you and food. The dieter's diary is a four star aid for behavior modification. Its goal is to teach you to become master of your eating habits and to do that, first you must know what those habits are.

The ideal food diary is both an *eating* record and a *feeling* record. You list what you eat, the time you eat, with whom, and how you feel about what you eat – on a daily basis. This will give you a wealth of information about yourself that you can use for a wide range of personal fitness goals.

SAMPLE DIETER'S FOOD DIARY

Food	Amount Servings	Who I Ate With	Time	My Moods & Feelings	Calorie Total
					Input

What Your Food Diary Can Do For You

1. It makes you aware of what you're actually eating, not what you think you're eating. Everyone makes mistakes when they try to remember their day's intake, even undereaters. Your diary provides an accurate record to use for a variety of problem-solving issues.
2. It takes the "guilt" out of your personal evaluation. The simple act of recording your daily food intake objectifies the situation. You don't have to keep that neon sign "I ate cake" in your head all day. It's on paper, where you can see it more objectively, like a scientist viewing food.
3. It's a personalized dietary analysis, and a bargain at that! It shows you the quality of food you eat. You can use this to compare with the quality of food you should be eating in the food groups.
4. It records your eating patterns:
   - Your preference for certain foods
   - Times of day or days of the week you eat most often
   - food cues that get to you

5. It shows you your weak points and strong points. You can use these for habit change.
6. It reveals the emotions and feelings that you equate with food. You can use this to understand more about you, and find substitutes to feed your emotional needs.
7. It's a personal weight control monitor. You can use your diary for feedback to adjust your food intake when you find yourself gaining weight.

Many people lose weight simply by keeping a diary and using it to improve their food intake and eating habits. But keep in mind that a diary isn't a *menu* or *meal plan.* A diary is what you actually eat, even with a menu or meal plan in front of you. Be completely honest in your record keeping. It's your record for you. The better your record, the better your progress and self-evaluation.

How To Use Your Diary

Pre-Diet Diary. This diary is used to target problem areas. You list your regular food intake when you are acting normally. You write down everything you eat – no cheating – including the fluids you drink. It's best to keep this diary for two weeks before a diet, since that will give you a realistic picture of your average intake and eating patterns on week days and weekends. Using Food Group recommendations for dieters, you can compare what you've been eating to what you should be eating and plug in the gaps to create a balanced, slenderizing food plan. You can study your eating patterns, moods and feelings to use as guides to problem areas that need resolution.

During Diet Diary. This diary can be used to track your progress, to keep you in line and as a self-monitoring tool. Keep this diary for the first four weeks of your diet, then one day a week as a checkpoint. Every so often, keep a weekly record again to see if fat foods are creeping in, your protein is up to par, and you're getting enough fiber, calcium and water. In addition, you can see how your eating habits are improving.

Failsafe Maintenance. This diary can be used to keep you at ideal weight for life. If you see yourself gaining more than five pounds (five pounds can be water weight), keep a diary for a week and evaluate what happened. By maintenance, you will be so knowledgeable about your intake and eating habits, you'll be able to take action in a snap. *See* Maintenance

◆ **DIARY, EXERCISE** A daybook of activity. The story of you and your energy output. The exercise diary should be tacked on to your food diary for the best effect. But many people have a difficult time with food, and while food is becoming more controllable, it might be best to keep your exercise diary separate. Its goal is to get you moving, and keep you moving on a regular basis.

Since most overweight people have a tendency to resist exercise, your exercise diary is both a record of your aerobic activity and your feelings before, during and after it. This will give you feedback you can use to develop an effective program for yourself. You record the exercise you did, the amount of time you did it, where, and how you felt about it. You can use this as a gauge to find a comfortable place to exercise, to choose exercises that please you (so you'll keep doing them), and to release your resistance on paper. Also include your average Daily Activity level, since this burns calories too.

The Ideal Dieter's Diary

Both diaries combined – food and exercise – make the ideal weight loss record. If you keep a combined record from the first day of your diet, tracking your food and insuring that you exercise three times each week, you get four stars for successful dieting. Your diary will be your best diet ally and a fabulous support system. It provides diet, exercise, feelings, behavior and self monitoring in one EZ system.

SAMPLE EXERCISE DIARY

Aerobic Choice	Minutes Performed	Moods & Feelings	General Daily Activity	Gen. Cal Burned	Total Cal Burned
				Aerobic Cal Burn	______ Output

NOTE: Notice the column on the far right of your diaries. When you keep a combined diary, and add up the calories you ate each day, and the calories you burned with exercise, you can track your progress like an athlete.

▲ **DIETARY ANALYSIS** a review and rating of your average food intake. There are four steps to making a dietary analysis:

1. Recording what you actually eat
2. Adding up the nutrient value of what you eat
3. Comparing your nutrient intake with recommended daily nutrient intake (RDAs)
4. Filling in the missing gaps in your diet. This might mean adding some foods, while subtracting others, not simply adding in the missing nutrients.

Dietary analyses are best when prepared by a registered dietitian, because they have all the information for nutrient calculations in their heads or on floppy disks. This makes an extremely complicated process seem easy. In addition, they can make on-the-spot evaluations, and personal recommendations from speaking with you, reviewing the outward signs of your physical health. In a sense, in a 1/2 hour dietary analysis with an RD, you are getting ten years and 1/2 hour's worth of education, and you're only paying for the half hour.

Standard dietary analyses don't include behaviors and moods, which is a big part of your eating idiosyncrasies. What you eat is often contingent on how you feel and how you react when you face situations like stress. If you change what you eat, without changing your headset about eating, old habits creep in and one day, you find you're eating for weight gain again.

➡ How To Make A Dietary Analysis

Record what you eat for one week.

The Long Way: Use our calorie counter which gives you protein, fat, and carbohydrate levels, along with calories. You can tally your nutrient intake (using the calorie counter) then compare your intake to the recommended levels in ● Diets.

The Short Way: Skip the endless calculations and compare your servings of meats, dairy, fruits, vegetables and grains to the recommended servings in Food Groups. Plug in the servings in food groups that you are not eating, and take out the servings in food groups you are overeating. You have an excellent analysis and solution in a snap.

● **DIETARY GUIDELINES** A fundamental set of standards for nutrition and health from the U.S. Department of Agriculture and the U.S. Department of Health and Human Services. First issued in 1980, these guidelines cite six areas for concern in your daily diet, and one major health concern as the second point – "Maintain Your Ideal Weight." If you're a part of the population (more than 1/4) who has to get to ideal weight, before you can think about maintaining it, you might not think these guidelines apply to you. Look again! The other six guidelines set the example for a very healthy diet for weight loss and maintenance.

The seven standards are:

1. Eat a Variety of Foods (from the basic food groups)
2. Maintain Ideal Weight
3. Avoid too much fat, saturated fat, and cholesterol
4. Eat foods with adequate starch and fiber (carbohydrates)
5. Avoid too much sugar
6. Avoid too much sodium
7. If you drink alcohol, do so in moderation.

If you use the six food guidelines as the basis of your daily diet, you'll gradually lose weight, and be in good shape to maintain it. But many people say the guidelines are too general. They were intended to be that way. Every year, researchers come closer to finding more exact information that explains what "too much" or "adequate" means for weight loss, maintenance and health. The government simply weighed in on the safe side, confining itself to guidelines that adhered to the Hippocratic oath, *First Do No Harm.* If more commercial diets followed that principle, we'd be seeing less weight regain. You might add two extras to the list of standards to boost your fitness results: 8. Exercise regularly, and 9. Drink plenty of water daily. *See* Food Groups for more specific guidelines. And ● topics.

DIETS, WEIGHT LOSS Calorie restricted diets that result in weight loss. The key to remember with calorie restricted diets is WHAT KIND OF WEIGHT LOSS? All weight loss is not created equal. The weight you want to lose is FAT. The weight you *do not want to lose* is MUSCLE. The weight you want to balance is WATER.

When you lose muscle, you regain your weight after your diet phase is over. Why diet if you are going to gain your weight back because of the kind of diet you chose?

There is a simple sliderule you can use to determine if a diet is going to provide fat loss or muscle losses.

BALANCED DIETS provide fat loss.

UNBALANCED DIETS provide muscle losses (and fat loss) especially very low calorie diets (VLCDs) for rapid weight loss..

How can you determine if a diet is not balanced? Compare the foods used in the diet to the foods required daily in the Food Groups. (See Food Groups.) This will give you a very easy way to rate commercial diets to insure that you are paying for a proper program. If the diet does not include all of the food groups, it is not balanced.

There are certain circumstances which require unbalanced diets, such as diabetes, since the person cannot metabolize carbohydrates. But this condition is a metabolic disorder that requires the care of a physician; therefore, it is a different issue than the ones facing average dieters.

Guide To Dieting

If you are obese and have no other medical complications, your doctor would most likely recommend a food group plan as the diet of first choice. Anything less will not be the best for you.

If you are overweight, your diet of first choice should not be one that provides less than 1000 calories per day (women) and less than 1400 calories per day (men). They allow you to lose muscle.

If you go on a very low calorie diet for rapid weight loss, or an imbalanced diet, you can wind up fatter than you started, and have greater hunger after the diet is over — hunger that wasn't present before the diet. Your weight gain will be rounder all over. You can face bouts of binge eating that were not part of your life before the diet.

The diet you choose for weight loss is one of the most important choices of your life. You are investing your body, time, energy, health, money, and emotions. You are not just investing your extra weight.

The *best and most lasting* form of weight loss is achieved with the following diet components:

REAL FOOD
BALANCED FOOD GROUPS — LEAN VERSION
HEALTHY CALORIE LEVELS:
  WOMEN 1000-1500
  MEN 1400-1800
EXERCISE

Believe it or not, dieting is not as complicated as you've been told. Learning how to eat a healthy, balanced diet is the complicated part, especially for dieters who have been trained to eat oddly by unbalanced diets. But once you make the shift, you have it as a healthy skill for life. Make the next diet you choose a healthy, balanced one. That way, you build yourself up on a diet, rather than break down.

Types of Diets

FADS *See* Fads.
FASTS *See* Fasting. Undereating.
FRUIT *See* Fruit Diet.
HIGH PROTEIN *See* Protein. Liquid Protein Diets.
KETOGENIC *See* Ketones. Ketogenic Diets.
LOW OR NO CARBOHYDRATE *See* Ketogenic Diets.
MODIFIED FAST *See* Ketogenic Diets.
POWDERED PROTEIN *See* Supplements.
PROTEIN SPARING MODIFIED FAST *See* PSMF.
RAPID WEIGHT LOSS *See* Rapid Weight Loss.
STARVATION *See* Starvation.
VEGETABLE, VEGETARIAN *See* Protein. Food Groups.
VERY LOW CALORIE DIET *See* VLCD.

DIGESTION

O Gastric Juice Producers

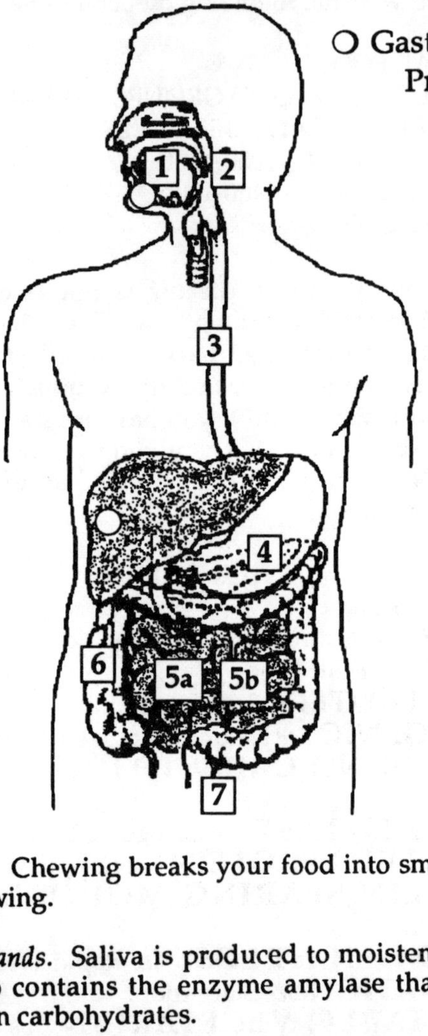

1 MOUTH Chewing breaks your food into smaller pieces for swallowing.

O *Salivary Glands.* Saliva is produced to moisten your food. Saliva also contains the enzyme amylase that begins to break down carbohydrates.

2 PHARYNX The food goes to your pharynx by your voluntary motion. After this point, peristalsis takes over. Peristalsis is a slow, wavelike motion that moves food through your entire digestive tract.

3 **Esophagus** Peristalsis pushes food through your esophagus into your stomach

4 **Stomach (Mid-Section) 1-4 Hours** Food mixes with gastric juices in your stomach. They include water, hydrochloric acid and the enzyme that begins to break down protein. A semi-liquid mass called Chyme is formed. Peristalsis pushes the Chyme out of your stomach into your small intestines.

5a **Small Intestines** When Chyme enters your small intestines, your pancreas secretes digestive juices that include acid-neutralizers. If fats are present, bile is secreted from your Gallbladder. Bile separates fats into droplets to prepare them for reaction with pancreatic enzymes. These chemical reactions convert food into nutrients that can be absorbed by your blood. The remainder of the Chyme goes into your Large Intestine.

❍ Your Liver produces bile acids that store in your gallbladder for use in fat breakdown in small intestines

❍ Your pancreas produces digestive juices and enzymes for additional carbohydrate and protein breakdown in small intestines.

5b **Absorption (From Small Intestines)** Nutrients pass into your bloodstream from your small intestines.

GLUCOSE (FROM CARBOHYDRATES)
FATTY ACIDS & GLYCEROL (FROM FATS)
AMINO ACIDS (FROM PROTEINS)
VITAMIN & MINERALS (WATER AND FAT SOLUBLE)
CHYME WITH LYMPH (AND OTHER SUBSTANCES)

6 **Large Intestines** Undigested Chyme (plus fiber) enters your large intestine where it absorbs water. Your large intestines have no enzymes, so no further digestion takes place.

7 **Rectum** After Chyme passes through your large intestine, it is excreted as waste.

DISEASES, weight-related. *See* Risks.

DIURETIC A medication that increases urine output, such as lasix or diazide. Diuretics are used for serious conditions and should not be confused with laxatives, which increase overall bowel excretion. Mild diuretics are often called water pills, but even these should not be used casually. Loss of body water can cause serious fluid imbalance and major disorders if prolonged. DIURETICS SHOULD NOT BE USED WITHOUT MEDICAL SUPERVISION.

DRUGS Prescription or non-prescription medications or aids. The excessive use of any drug causes depletion of essential nutrients from your body. Absorption is hampered, excretion of nutrients is increased, and appetite can be decreased, which adds to nutrient depletion since you are not replacing them in your daily diet. A dangerous combination is sleeping pills, use of stimulants and alcohol. It can start gradually, by taking stimulants as a diet aid, leading to sleeplessness and the need for sleep aids. Add alcohol to the mix and it can be deadly, since your system is constantly swinging up and down, and your perceptions and responses are altered. It's best to avoid over-the-counter drugs or diet aids, since they can often be a catalyst for use of other medications. Recommended therapy is to discontinue all non-prescription drugs and adhere to a balanced diet and exercise program, drinking plenty of water. If use is excessive, see your physician.

e

▲ **EATING** The process of acquiring energy you need for metabolism. In its ideal state, eating is a physiological process, but it can also be influenced by emotions, psychology, and environment. *See* Digestion. Metabolism. Appetite. Hunger.

▲ **EATING HABITS** Your eating style. How you eat, as opposed to what you eat. Patterns of eating. Your eating habits may play a greater role in weight gain than any other factor. They include your adult eating patterns and habits carried over from childhood, where you first learned about food. Often food is used for rewards or punishments in childhood, with desserts being withheld for punishment or proffered as rewards. No one can recall hearing: "I'm so proud of you. Here's a cup of fruit. " It's more like: "You can have a double scoop of ice cream tonight." This is how sweets and fats come to be regarded as the foods that give comfort or pleasure.

Eating habits are also cultural and ethnic, and many of your food cravings (emotional) center around family gatherings where everyone brings their favorite recipe and talks about old times. Food also has peer links. The foods your teenage friends perceived as "cool" (now "bad" meaning "good") are foods you can equate with being popular or fun; therefore *not eating* them makes you think you're dull or uncool.

The primary eating habits that lead to weight gain are:
EMOTIONAL EATING — using food to satisfy other needs you may have.

STRESS EATING — using food to soothe you when you are tense.

EATING ON THE RUN — eating too fast, which means you can eat more without being aware of it.

LATE NIGHT EATING — your metabolism is slower in the evening and it gets even slower in sleep. Late night food doesn't digest easily and more calories can store.

NOT EATING BREAKFAST — this is the first meal of the day to give you energy and fire up your metabolism. When you don't eat breakfast, your metabolism can be sluggish until noon.

SOCIAL EATING — feeling obligated to eat because everyone else is doing it.

RELYING ON SUGAR FOR ENERGY BOOSTS — sugar is empty calories and usually comes along with excess fat. This keeps you in a sugar/fat cycle that tends to take precedence over healthy foods.

The key to resolving your fat-promoting eating habits is to find rewards for yourself that are not food. You can substitute pleasurable non-food activities for your most common habit problems. A good way to keep yourself from falling into poor eating habits is to practice a regular program of relaxation or meditation every day. *See* Relaxation. Meditation.

ECTOMORPH. A body type that is characterized by a long thin linear look, symbolized by the column. *See* Body Type.

ENDOMORPH A body type that is characterized by roundness all over, symbolized by the circle. *See* Body Type.

ENERGY The heat of living and being active. Every process in your body generates heat. When you eat, it produces heat. When your body takes up the nutrients from food, it generates heat. The nutrients give you the energy you need to be alive and active, and the process of using that energy generates heat. This heat is measured in units, or calories. From this heat measurement, scientists were able to measure the nutrient density of foods and the energy effects of exercise, along with thousands of other substances and processes in the universe.

When you eat, the heat you produce should match the heat you give off. Eating is *INPUT* (taking in the nutrients). Movement and activity (including exercise) is *OUTPUT* (using those nutrients).

When your *INPUT* matches your *OUTPUT*, you are at ideal weight. Overweight(obesity) and dieting are not balanced energy states. In overweight and obesity, your *OUTPUT* is less than your *INPUT*, and in dieting, it's intentionally reversed— your *OUTPUT* exceeds your *INPUT*. We put this in energy wheels for you in each of these states. *See* Obesity, for the energy wheels.

▲ **ENERGY EXPENDITURE** Output. The amount of calories you burn daily. *See* Exercise.

ENZYMES Chemicals that can break down other chemicals without being changed themselves. There are dozens of enzymes involved in digestion and metabolism of your food. Each one can only act on a specific nutrient, and no other. In digestion alone, there are 3 enzymes for carbohydrates, 6 for protein, and 1 for fat. During digestion, these enzymes split the molecules of carbohydrates, proteins and fats into smaller molecules in each part of digestion from your mouth through your small intestines, where absorption finally takes place. Gastric juices in your stomach stimulate the release of hormones, which in turn stimulate the release of enzymes. It's a chain reaction that keeps on splitting molecules into smaller and smaller forms, until they wind up in the form that can be absorbed by your blood. Carbohydrates become glucose, proteins become amino acids, and fats become fatty acids and glycerol. From your blood, they go to your cells where a whole new series of enzymes activate the chemical reactions of metabolism.

This entire process starts all over again with each meal. That's what's known as enzyme — catalyzed reactions.Diets that claim that they catalyze important enzyme reactions that burn fat are only talking about the natural process of digestion and metabolism that your body does automatically. So you're paying for what you've already got. *See* Digestion and Metabolism.

EPINEPHRINE A hormone produced by your adrenal glands that reduces hunger by stimulating the release of glucose from your liver. When your blood glucose levels rise, hunger is abated (in your brain). Exercise increases the production of epinephrine, which is one of the reasons why it decreases your appetite.

The Epinepherine Effect

Have you ever had a "shaky" feeling, where you can literally feel tremors inside, and weak even though you just ate. That's the epinepherine effect.

It's caused by eating too much sugar.

If you wake in the morning and have orange juice, pancakes and sugary syrup, and the pancake mix has added sugar, you can experience the epinepherine effect. Your sugar intake causes your blood glucose to shoot UP. Insulin is secreted to metabolize the glucose. Your blood sugar starts to drop quickly. Epinepherine is released which reacts on your liver to release glucose, and the shakes start. Rapid heartbeat, cold sweats, a feeling of sudden fear or dread — your body literally quakes inside.

To stop the effect, you need protein and sugar back to back — a 1/2 cup of orange juice and 1/2 cup of milk. The orange juice will stop the quick sugar drop and the protein will prolong digestion, stabilizing the effect.

If you had protein with a high carbohydrate breakfast in the first place, you wouldn't have the effect, and you'd be in great shape for weight loss.

▲ **EUSTRESS** Good stress, specifically the good stress of exercise. Exercise is stress, but it's a beneficial stress, meeting a challenge and overcoming it. The benefits are the opposite of negative stress, *after* you complete the exercise. You see a lower heart rate, lower blood pressure, soothed respiration. That's why it's important to do the required 20-30 minutes of an aerobic exercise. It's the time needed to create those after-exercise effects. If you break earlier, you can be in the midpoint of stress, and feel tenser as a result. The part that is not computed is the feeling of wellbeing that you get from meeting that challenge and mastering it. It gives you a sense of confidence and pride that shines from within.

EXCHANGE LIST Energy equivalents. Exchange lists are a system that allows foods in one food group to be substituted for foods in another group for therapeutic use, such as diets for diabetes (since the diabetic has trouble metabolizing carbohydrates) or in lactose-allergy diets, where the person has trouble digesting milk. The exchange list indicates the other sources of energy which can replace those foods, while still providing equal nutritional value.

The term *exchange list* is sometimes used in weight loss diets to refer to foods in the same food group that can be used in place of another food in that group to achieve similar energy, while being similarly low fat (for preference). Or it can cross groups, as in a vegetarian's diet for weight loss, which would have to provide alternate sources of protein, instead of animal sources.

▲ **EXCUSES** Reasons why you think you can't accomplish something. They're simply attitudes, and you can change them. *See* Rationalizations.

◆ **EXERCISE** Motion. Dynamic Action. The motion in exercise sets off chemical reactions in your body that use nutrients and produce heat as a byproduct.

There are two forms of exercise, aerobic and anaerobic, named after the type of energy that is used for each form.

First it is important to know that the chemical in your body that acts as the energy carrier for ALL PROCESSES, is called ATP — Adenosine TriPhosphate. It's made by a chemical called ADP — Adenosine DiPhosphate. When you eat food, the molecules are broken down into smaller forms. When the bonds of your food molecules are broken, energy escapes and some is captured by the bonds of ADP, and stored in the bonds of ATP. ATP travels around your body bringing energy to every part. When your heart beats, it means that a bond of ATP has been broken to provide energy. If you run down the stairs, bonds of ATP are being broken to provide the needed energy. When you exercise, the source of your energy is ATP. To break the bonds of ATP, OXYGEN is necessary.

AEROBIC EXERCISE. The source of energy for aerobic exercise is ATP and oxygen. The bonds of ATP break with oxygen, and supply glucose and fatty acids for fuel. This is your muscles' *preferred* form of energy. The supply of ATP is greater with aerobic exercise, and at first your circulation can't keep up with your activity if you burst into aerobic exercise too quickly. If you are a jogger, for instance, you walk first before you run, so that your circulation can pick up and supply more ATP, that will be needed for your aerobic workout. The entire aerobic workout is sustained on ATP and oxygen (providing fuel).

ANAEROBIC EXERCISE. The source of energy for anaerobic exercise is different. It's ATP without oxygen to break the bonds. Since you burst into action without warming up and increasing your circulation, your body has to make ATP without sufficient oxygen. This is called the GLYCOLYTIC METHOD, meaning that your body uses glucose and glycogen to make ATP. This process produces LACTIC ACID along with the ATP. Lactic levels that accumulate to critical levels result in *fatigue.* There is a limit to the amount of ATP that your body can make anaerobically. If you burst into a run with your muscles tensed up, and you aren't breathing deeply, you can use up your anaerobic ATP and not get enough oxygen to produce aerobic ATP, and you can collapse from exhaustion. Lactic acid levels to excess (ketones) can be toxic.

Sudden, spontaneous motion that is sustained is not the way to start exercising aerobically. Under ordinary circumstances, if you burst into exercise with anaerobic ATP, part of the way into your activity, your aerobic ATP will catch up, and start being manufactured with the necessary oxygen. But dieters circumstances aren't ordinary. They are restricting their calories. And if you're on a diet that is restricting its carbohydrates (the primary muscle fuel), you're producing a high level of ketones to begin with. Sudden, spontaneous exercise on a no or low carbohydrate diet could be dangerous.

It's one more reason you should think ten times before you go on an imbalanced diet.

Anaerobic energy use is something that trained athletes deal with as a part of training. Mile runners, for instance, start with a sudden anaerobic burst, and the speed of the run is so stressful, that the aerobic ATP never gets a chance to catch up. They learn to gauge their point of exhaustion, and using this, they have to meter their anaerobic ATP, or they could collapse from fatigue. But athletes eat sound, balanced diets to achieve this ability.

You should too. Eat plenty of carbohydrates daily, in case you need sudden and sustained energy in a crisis situation. It's your body's best protection.

Why You Need To Exercise

To fine-tune your metabolism. Calorie restriction can reduce your calorie-burning power by causing your metabolic rate to drop as much as 10-15%. You can burn fewer calories, even though you cut them to burn more. This could cause you to stop losing weight or to lose very slowly. Exercise raises your metabolic rate by 10-15% to offset this loss of burning power.

To preserve your muscle: Fat is the only loss you can afford on a diet. Muscle losses undermine your metabolism and reduce your burning power. Exercise preserves muscle during a diet, to insure that you burn only fat.

To balance your body composition. At the end of your diet, your fat-to-muscle status is of primary concern. It will determine how many calories you can eat at maintenance without gaining weight. Studies showed that two people of the same height, weight, and sex can eat the same number of calories at the end of a diet, and one will gain while the other will not. Why? The one who won't gain has a low-fat/high muscle body.

To gain oxygen for fat burn. When you exercise, you use more oxygen. For fat to be burned, oxygen is necessary. With aerobic exercise, you can expect greater burn of stored fat.

To increase intestinal motility. Food passes through your intestines better when exercise is a regular routine. An average nonexerciser can take 24 hours to complete one digestive cycle, an obese nonexerciser can take up to 48 hours. Too slow! Food that lingers in your intestines can stagnate and lead to digestive disorders or increase your risk of bowel cancer. Exercise speeds food transit time through your intestines. Athletes show intestinal motility of 4 to 6 hours to complete digestion.

To regulate your appetite. Loss of appetite follows a good workout. When activity levels are low, studies show that people increase their calorie intake.

To fight anxiety and depression. Endorphins are opiatelike chemicals produced in your brain that modulate pain and moods. Exercise increases their production, leaving you with a euphoric feeling. Your circulation is improved and this creates a sense of well-being. Therapists are beginning to prescribe aerobic exercise and dance as therapy against anxiety and depression, with one study boasting an 82 percent success rate in hard-to-treat patients.

To reduce stress. 50 to 75% of all organic illnesses are aggravated by or related to stress. Stress stimulates your sympathetic nervous system, speeding your heart rate, increasing your blood pressure, and contributing to cardiovascular disease. Exercise reverses the stress response by reducing your heart rate, lowering your blood pressure, and improving your sense of control.

To lose fat for disease prevention. High body fat has been linked to most of our major lifestyle diseases, including hypertension, heart disease, diabetes, and cancer — specifically colon cancer in men and breast cancer in women. Since exercise reduces body fat, you reduce the risk of acquiring these diseases by exercising. Recent studies show that exercise can significantly reduce the risk of heart attack by improving heart and lung function and increasing the concentration of HDL (good cholesterol).

To increase your energy output. Movement requires energy. The more you move, the more energy you use, which means more calories burned.

In addition to its metabolic benefits, exercise is the best *behavior substitute* for eating.

HEALTH BENEFITS OF EXERCISE

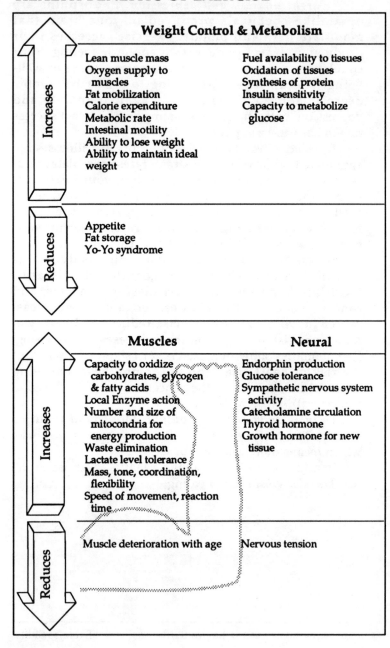

Weight Control & Metabolism

Increases

- Lean muscle mass
- Oxygen supply to muscles
- Fat mobilization
- Calorie expenditure
- Metabolic rate
- Intestinal motility
- Ability to lose weight
- Ability to maintain ideal weight
- Fuel availability to tissues
- Oxidation of tissues
- Synthesis of protein
- Insulin sensitivity
- Capacity to metabolize glucose

Reduces

- Appetite
- Fat storage
- Yo-Yo syndrome

Muscles

Increases

- Capacity to oxidize carbohydrates, glycogen & fatty acids
- Local Enzyme action
- Number and size of mitocondria for energy production
- Waste elimination
- Lactate level tolerance
- Mass, tone, coordination, flexibility
- Speed of movement, reaction time

Reduces

- Muscle deterioration with age

Neural

Increases

- Endorphin production
- Glucose tolerance
- Sympathetic nervous system activity
- Catecholamine circulation
- Thyroid hormone
- Growth hormone for new tissue

Reduces

- Nervous tension

RECOMMENDED DOSE — **AEROBIC (LOW IMPACT)**
3 X per week, 30 min session

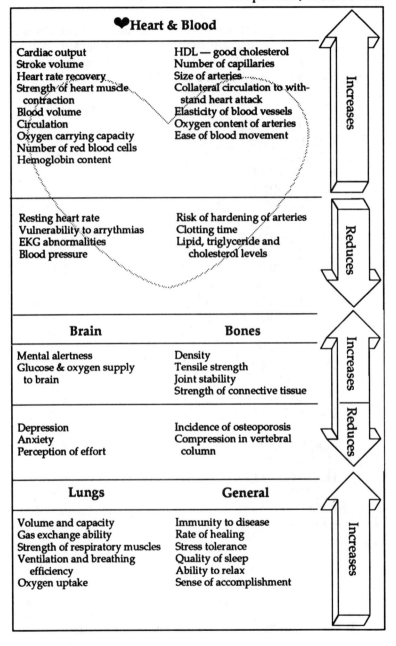

❤Heart & Blood

Increases

Cardiac output	HDL — good cholesterol
Stroke volume	Number of capillaries
Heart rate recovery	Size of arteries
Strength of heart muscle contraction	Collateral circulation to withstand heart attack
Blood volume	Elasticity of blood vessels
Circulation	Oxygen content of arteries
Oxygen carrying capacity	Ease of blood movement
Number of red blood cells	
Hemoglobin content	

Reduces

Resting heart rate	Risk of hardening of arteries
Vulnerability to arrythmias	Clotting time
EKG abnormalities	Lipid, triglyceride and cholesterol levels
Blood pressure	

Brain / Bones

Increases

Brain	Bones
Mental alertness	Density
Glucose & oxygen supply to brain	Tensile strength
	Joint stability
	Strength of connective tissue

Reduces

Brain	Bones
Depression	Incidence of osteoporosis
Anxiety	Compression in vertebral column
Perception of effort	

Lungs / General

Increases

Lungs	General
Volume and capacity	Immunity to disease
Gas exchange ability	Rate of healing
Strength of respiratory muscles	Stress tolerance
Ventilation and breathing efficiency	Quality of sleep
Oxygen uptake	Ability to relax
	Sense of accomplishment

CALORIE BURN FOR EXERCISE AND ACTIVITIES

The average calorie burn for exercise and activities is based on 150 pound adults. If you weigh less than that, you will burn a little less than the levels shown here. If you weigh more, you will burn a little more.

	CALS/HR
AEROBIC DANCE	445
BADMINTON	350
BASEBALL	280
BASKETBALL	750
BED MAKING	210
BICYCLING	415
BOWLING	190
CALISTHENICS	415
CANOEING	300
CAR WASHING	230
CARPENTRY	305
COOKING	100
CROSS COUNTRY SKI	700
DANCING	250
DESK WORK	100
DISHWASHING	135
DOWNHILL SKIING	595
DRIVING	100
EATING	90
FLOOR WASHING	250
FOOTBALL	600
GARDENING	390
HIKING HILLS	600
ICE HOCKEY	900
JOGGING	655
LACROSSE	900

	CALS/HR
MARTIAL ARTS	790
MOWING LAWN (REG)	460
MOWING (POWER)	270
PAINTING (WALLS)	165
READING	90
RIDING A HORSE	415
ROWING	648
RUNNING IN PLACE	510
RUNNING (POWER)	800
SAILING	155
SHOPPING	165
SKATING	350
SKIPPING ROPE	510
SLEEPING	65
SNOW SHOVELING	610
SOCCER	600
SQUARE DANCING	420
SQUASH	775
SWIMMING	300
SWIMMING (POWER)	600
TABLE TENNIS	300
TENNIS	425
VOLLEYBALL	350
WALKING (BRISK)	255
WALKING (POWER)	345
WATCHING TV	80
WEIGHT LIFTING	300
WINDOW WASHING	250
WRITING	90
YOGA	230

f

FAD A diet or diet-related aid that is popular for a brief time, even though it may not be healthy, safe, or do what it promises. Fad diets play on your vulnerability as a person with weight problems, luring you with claims that equal your secret desires: Fat Melts Like Magic! Miracle Food Removes Fat! Secret Formula Makes You Slim Overnight! Some fads like liquid protein diets were downright dangerous, and others like patches were harmless as pet rocks. But even a harmless fad isn't worth the price of emotional setbacks. You want to believe it will work, you try it believing, and your spirit takes a beating when weight loss fails again. The best way to combat the lure of fad diets is to consider the investment you're making – your body, health, money, pride, self esteem – then get all the facts you can about dieting safely, and compare the risks. You'll probably find that safe dieting is the secret formula you've been looking for all along. *See* Food Groups

FAMILY TENDENCIES Your pre-disposition for obesity based on genetic and *trained* factors. Scientists have not been able to determine what part of overweight or obesity is exclusively a matter of genes, and how much is a matter of conditioning, or childhood training. Childhood eating patterns carry over into adulthood as part of the family tendency picture. Therefore, the following figures represent both aspects:

If you have 1 overweight parent – you are 30% more likely to be overweight.

If you have 2 overweight parents – you are 70% more likely to be overweight.

Studies of adopted children support the "learned" aspects of obesity as a major factor. Adopted children tend to display the same incidence of obesity as their unrelated brothers and sisters. However, the older the adopted child, the less likely these tendencies became, which suggests that overweight habits are learned at a very early age. On the plus side of the picture, learned behaviors can be unlearned, or changed. Changing your eating patterns (carried over from childhood) is one of the purposes of behavior modification. *See* Eating Habits.

● **FAST FOOD** Food you can buy quickly and eat quickly, usually processed and non-nutritious. And fattening.

You don't have to give up fast foods on a diet. Make your own variety in low-fat stews, casseroles, pasta salads and soups that you freeze and reheat, or microwave in a snap.

With a little detective work, you can find healthy fast foods in the neighborhood near your job, so you're not caught in the drive-through window of a processed food palace because you need a quick lunch. Many restaurants and supermarkets have salad bars with lite dressings, and most delis have barbecued chickens (you can remove the skin). Make eating out an adventure, rather than an exercise in denial. Have fun finding slim foods in local eateries and keep your own restaurant guide. But change one feature about fast foods, don't eat them fast! People who have a slower rate of eating stay slimmer.

FASTING Going without food. *See* Starvation.

● **FAT, FOOD** Concentrated energy. One gram of fat gives you 9 calories, twice the amount in protein or carbohydrates. You need some fat in your body for insulation, support, and protection of your organs, and to act as a carrier for the fat-soluble vitamins A, D, E, and K, aiding in their absorption.

Fat supplies essential fatty acids, including linoleic acid, which is needed for proper growth in children, to maintain cell membranes and regulate cholesterol metabolism, and to prevent drying and flaking of the skin. But how much fat do you need?

Studies show that 1 tablespoon of corn oil — rich in linoleic acid — provides all the essential fat needed by most people. The rest is extra fat and it arrives in a form that stores easily in your body.

The average American derives 40-45 percent of his or her calories from fat. In fat intake studies of 35- to 40-year olds, only 13 percent of the males and 17 percent of the females had a fat intake of less than 35 percent of their total calories. Over a third had a fat intake providing 45 percent or more of their total calories.

Dietary trends over the last decade indicate that our total intake of calories is down, so why are we still fat? Our fat consumption is up. We are eating more fat packed into fewer calories.

When you keep your diet low in fat, the results are dynamic. You feel a cleaner, lighter system in the absence of excess fat. You begin to notice the flavor and subtle tastes of other foods that you may not have appreciated before, because your taste buds were blunted by your desire for the taste and texture of fat.

FAT, BODY Lipid stores. There are 2 types of fat in your body, white fat and brown fat. White fat is the most prevalent form of fat, but the least active body tissue. Brown Fat is a small percent of your total body fat (usually 1%), but it is metabolic active, meaning it is more related to burning energy than storing. *See* Brown Fat.

FAT CELLS storehouses for fat. Also called adipose tissue.

There are two kinds of fat cells in your body:
Hypertrophic — oversized cells filled with fat
Hyperplastic — normal-sized cells in greater numbers

The nutrients left over after metabolism that were not needed for body maintenance and repair, and not burned off with activity and exercise — store in your fat cells as lipids. When you accumulate a higher-than-normal level of lipid storage, you have obesity.

In infancy, your fat cells grow primarily by increasing their number, not their size. The number of cells you produce can range from 2 to 5 times the normal number. At some undetermined point in adolescence, the production of new cells slows down, and weight gain increases the size of cells. Cell size can range from 2 to 5 times the normal size.

Adult-onset obesity is associated with hypertrophic cells — fatter fat cells.

Infant or adolescent onset obesity is associated with hyperplastic cells — more normal sized cells.

Both types of cells exist in most people, but more hypertrophic cells exist in obese people, or people who have been obese and have lost weight. It is assumed that excess weight gain in infancy and childhood causes overproduction of these fatter fat cells, and prevention of childhood weight gain will limit their production. The thinner you are younger, the less fat cells you will have in adulthood, making it easier to stay slim.

Losing weight can shrink the size of cells, but not their number. Until liposuction surgery, there was no known way to change the number of fat cells in your body. By removing fat cells, liposuction alters this phenomenon. However, it does not change the fact that remaining cells can increase in size. This means that weight gain after liposuction will appear in isolated areas, swelling existing fat cells to a greater size. The result is unevenly distributed fat, or pockets of fat in formerly non-fat areas. Men have been found to deposit fat in the breast area, after liposuction for midriff and abdominal fat. Women can deposit fat in their upper bodies, when they were formerly lower-body fat distributors. Existing cells don't change their location or spread out over a larger area after removal of some cells. They stay where they are and fat goes to the areas where cells are. Losses of blood can be extensive in fat cell removal. As a result, cell removal isn't recommended as weight loss therapy. Shrinking the size of the cells by shrinking the fat content of the diet is the best fat cell therapy to date.

FAT DISTRIBUTION Where fat predominates. Primary fat sites. Where you deposit your fat is an important issue to consider, since fat sites influence health risks. Two types of fat distribution have been classified as the primary ways you deposit fat.

Upper Body Fat	Lower Body Fat
The common sites are neck, back, abdomen, waist, upper hips	The common sites are hips,thighs, stomach, calves to ankles
Predominates in men	Predominates in women
Predominates in men with diabetes	More common after menopause
Also seen in women with diabetes	Not linked to disease
More common in smokers	Harder to lose
Linked to heart disease	
Easier to lose	

Either sex can deposit fat in upper or lower body, but the crossover is more common in women. Upper body fat distributors are the ones who should be more concerned about losing weight, since it increases your risk of heart disease and diabetes. for example, obese people in general have 3 times the risk of acquiring diabetes, but obese people who are upper body fat distributors have 10 times the risk of diabetes.

Since liposuction surgery can lead to fat distribution in areas of the body where fat didn't predominate before, it is an issue for women who think it is harmless to remove fat cells from their hips and thighs. If it changes you from a lower body fat distributor to an upper body depositor, it will make the fat that you carry more risky.

▲ **FAT EYES** A behavioral term for seeing yourself fatter than you are, after losing weight.

Many people who have carried weight for a long time, have difficulty seeing themselves without that weight around them. In a sense, they wear a shadow of their old fat. This can cause a diet relapse, and steps must be taken to own your new leaner self. Weight is often seen as strength or power to a person who has carried it, and thin can seem weak or vulnerable. Often, diets that cause rapid weight loss can foster this image problem, because the physical changes occur too fast and there isn't time for adjustment to the new, slim image. This is one of the reasons why thin/within imagery is so vital during a diet. Your thinner self is claimed in your mind, and you are more familiar with the sight and feeling of being slimmer when you arrive there. Any change in your outer appearance should be accompanied by supportive work on your inner view of yourself, since that makes the change ring true. *See* Imagery. Body Image. Mirror Exercises.

FAT TOOTH Desire for fats. The shadow behind your sweet tooth. The phenomenon of fat tooth emerged from studies on taste-preference at Rockefeller University. Normal weight college students were given a variety of mixtures of sugar and fat, and asked to rate them. Their findings showed:

Heavy cream solutions (37% fat) and 8% sugar were rated as pleasant.

When the sugar content was increased to 10%, the rating was *not* pleasant.

When the fat content was increased to 52% with 9% sugar, the mixture got the *highest* rating.

These studies suggest that a preference for fat may be hiding behind the desire for sugar. A higher fat mixture can increase your tolerance for sweets. On the reverse side of the coin, decreasing your fats can lead to a decrease in your tolerance of sugar. That means two problems can be solved for the price of one.

FAT-TO-MUSCLE RATIO Body composition. The proper proportion of body fat and muscle. *See Scale.*

FATIGUE Exhaustion. This can be brought on by nutrient deficiency on an imbalanced diet, or it can be the result of anaerobic exercise. Prolonged fatigue can be caused by a medical disorder and needs your doctor's care.

FATTY ACIDS The nutrients derived from fats, used by your body for energy. *See* Digestion.

▲ **FEAR OF FAILURE** An obstacle-course of feelings. Fear is an emotion that sets barriers up in front of you, whether those barriers are real or emotional. It is natural to feel fear about change, and weight loss is change, especially for a person who carries a great deal of weight.

It is also natural to fear failure if you have a history of rapid weight loss dieting, which led to rapid weight regain. Or you can fear the person who might emerge from the process, because you aren't familiar with that person; you're familiar with weight. You may have a spouse who would feel threatened by changes in your attitude and lifestyle, and this can generate fear. Or you may have an issue with expectations.

Setting unrealistic expectations is one of the biggest reasons for failure with weight loss. For instance, you've been overweight for several years, but you want to lose your weight in eight weeks. That's an unrealistic expectation, especially if you are more than 20% over your ideal weight, AND have used very low calorie diets in the past. However, this expectation — or desire — will send you to a diet that says "Lose 30 pounds in two months." That diet might be able to provide what it promises, but it will starve you and deprive you to do it. If you hang in for the duration and lose your weight, you'll gain it back, because you lost too much muscle tissue. You will think you're a failure, when it was the diet that failed you. You're left with the residue. The next time around, you fear what you're trying to do.

To deal with these issues, first you have to re-define failure. Then you have to plan how to deal with fear.

When you set a goal and try to achieve it, that's a success-minded attitude. If you fail to achieve it, that isn't failure. The effort is the achievement. "Failure" is an illusion, or imaginary monster. It will remain in front of you like an obstacle, until you kick it out of the room.

➡ How To Combat Fear of Failure

An excellent technique you can use is imagery to identify failure and how to get rid of it. This form of imagery is best done with a paper and pencil, instead of your mind, because you don't need any more pictures of failure in your mind. They can frighten you.

Take a notebook and write FAILURE in big letters on

the top of the page. Then draw something that comes to your mind to represent failure. It can be a stick figure, or a cartoon monster, or anything. Once you have your picture of FAILURE, you want to think of something that will remove it. For instance, if failure is a stick figure of some kind, draw yourself as a bigger stick figure with a broom, sweeping failure out of the picture. Or failure can be a black cloud and you can cross it out and draw a sun overhead. Draw as many pictures as you want, until you find the one that makes you laugh or feel better. Every time you think of failure, draw another picture of it and resolve the image.

Fear can be managed with relaxation exercises, especially the ones for meditation. In addition, you can change how you feel about fear by using the same formula as the one used for FAILURE. You can use this process for most of your obstacle-emotions and feelings. Back this up with positive self talk to replace negative self-talk, and you'll find you don't feel as much anxiety about trying again.

When you decide to try again, set healthy expectations. The way to prevent big gaps in your emotions from here to there, from overweight to ideal weight, is to use a step-goal approach. First lose ten pounds, then accept yourself at that place and with that thinner image. Then lose ten more pounds, and stabilize yourself. Use this approach to get to ideal weight.

● **FIBER** The undigestible part of plants. Also called roughage. The fact that fiber is undigestible means it doesn't get absorbed, or stored as fat. Most foods are broken down by digestive enzymes by the time they reach your intestines, but not fiber. It binds with water in your intestines, smoothing out bowel movements, preventing constipation and many digestive disorders. Where is fiber found? In complex carbohydrates.

FIBER AT A GLANCE

Recommended Diet Dose
25-35 grams/day
from the 5 Fibers

➡ 2 FIBERS AT EACH MEAL. INCLUDE ALL GROUPS

1 CELLULOSE

Bran · Whole Wheat Flour · Cabbage · Young Peas · Wax Beans · Green Beans · Brussel Sprouts · Apples · Broccoli · Peppers · Cuke Skins · Carrots

2 HEMI-CELLULOSE

Bran · Cereals · Whole Grains · Beet Root · Mustard Greens · Brussel Sprouts

❤ 3 GUMS

Oatmeal · Rolled Oat Products · Dried Beans

❤ 4 PECTIN

Apples · Squash · Citrus Fruits · Cauliflower · Cabbage · Carrots · Green Beans

❤ 5 LIGNIN

Bran · Cereals · Older Veggies · Green Beans · Strawberries · Pears · Radishes · Eggplant · Potatoes

CARBOHYDRATES

➡ 6 Servings Fiber Daily

Average Serving
Veg, Fruit, Cereal 1/2 Cup
Whole Fruit 1 small
Bread 1 Slice

Vitamin

Water 2 Qts Daily

Fiber binds with water. Drinking water keeps fiber from blocking.
Fiber binds w/trace minerals and can be excreted. Vit/min supplement.
➡ Increase fiber intake gradually over 2-8 weeks to prevent gas.

FIBER'S BENEFITS FOR DIETERS

Bonus To Dieters

- Fiber expands with water to fill your stomach, and fullness terminates hunger. Fullness also means a sense of satisfaction, and that's important when you're on a limited calorie program.
- Since fiber doesn't store as fat, you can use fiber foods to fill out a diet, so you don't feel deprived.
- Fiber-rich foods are lower in overall calories than non-fiber foods.
- Increased fiber intake leads to decreased intake of more fatty, sugary foods.
- Fiber foods take longer to chew, a very important habit to use to stay slim.
- Fiber increases your food transit time — the time it takes food to pass through your intestines. Faster transit time means less chance of food stagnation and calorie absorption. The longer food stays in your intestines, the more calories can be absorbed.

❤ • Fiber lowers your levels of bad cholesterol (LDL) without reducing good cholesterol (HDL).

- It stimulates bile flow from your liver and prevents bile absorption, which keeps gallstones from forming.
- It reduces intestinal pressure and allows food to be cleared from pouches that cause diverticulosis.
- It can help to prevent colon cancer by reducing bacteria that interact with fat and bile acids to create carcinogens. By moving stool more quickly, it prevents carcinogens from coming into contact with intestines.
- Gums in fibers are thought to delay emptying of the stomach and absorption of glucose, resulting in lower insulin levels in diabetics. It smoothes sugar surges.

▲ **FIGHT OR FLIGHT** The stress response. *See* Stress.

▲ **FOOD CUE** Something that triggers you to eat (other than mealtime). This can be a person, place, situation, event, or stimulus that causes you to reach for food on automatic pilot. Some of the most common food cues are:

- people in your family, or people who remind you of your family (where early eating patterns developed).
- places other than the kitchen or dining room where eating has been an accepted activity – eating in bed, in front of the TV, at movie theatres, at your desk in the office during breaks.
- situations which are emotionally charged, such as vacations, parties, family gatherings, weddings.
- events that cause stress, anxiety, fear or any strong emotion such as moving, a family illness, a job change.
- stimulus about food, such as pictures of food, food commercials, the refrigerator, kitchen, bakeries, supermarkets.

Here's how it happens:

1. You get the cue: You're making out your taxes. You owe more than you thought.
2. You feel an emotion (anxiety, frustration, depression).
3. To assuage that emotion, you eat.

➠ **How To Control Food Cues**

Food cue control is a study of action/reaction. Notice the typical "actions" that cause you to eat, then devise strategies that change your reaction to a non-food response, such as taking a walk, reading, working on a hobby, meditating. Your non-food reactions are called substitution behaviors, because you are replacing a bad habit with a good one. It helps to make a list of habits you find pleasurable and easy to do in a pinch, so you can arm yourself in advance with alternatives to food. The longer your list, the better equipped you'll be to conquer eating on cue.

food groups

The following pages 123-141 contain the Food Group section — a special feature for dieting smart. It gives you a complete food guide for healthy dieting and healthy eating the natural way.

You can use it to diet safely and achieve the fitness benefits you need for permanent weight maintenance. Or you can use it to insure that you're eating for nutritional fitness on a daily basis whether you are on a diet or off one. This is the foundation of health and power with food. You can use it for life.

● FOOD GROUPS The scientific system that sorts foods into groups according to the nutrients they yield (CALORIES). The nutrients that provide calories are Proteins, Carbohydrates, and Fats — and these calories are essential to your body for its growth, repair, maintenance and metabolism.

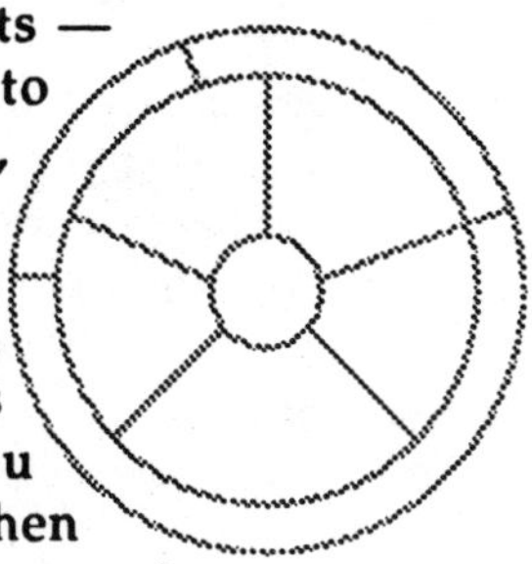

Eating for health means eating what the food groups recommend for essential energy. Eating less is not better for you, it leaves you deficient in your daily needs. When you are deficient, every body process is slightly altered to make up for these absences in nutrients. Over time, the mild alterations can turn into major imbalances. If you only make one change in your life, the best change you could make is to *eat everything in the food groups on a daily basis.* This applies to dieting also.

The easy way to deal with food is to start with the food groups as *the bottom line* every day. Think about your food life this way:

MY FIRST PRIORITY:
Eat Everything in the Food Groups Daily
MY SECOND PRIORITY:
Evaluate the Foods I Eat Beyond That

This makes your food life much simpler, especially on a diet.

When you are overweight and you begin eating everything in the food groups as the first priority, several benefits occur that begin to help you lose weight automatically. You are less hungry. You are getting fiber. You are more satisfied. You are getting all of your daily nutrients, vitamins, and minerals, and that makes everything work better, including your *metabolism.*

The food group system is the *most perfect diet* you can use for health or weight loss. And it's free! It's the science of food and metabolism.

➠ How To Diet with the Food Groups

The food group system is provided in energy wheels for easy use on a diet. When you choose all the lean varieties in the food groups, as shown in the wheels, you have the *most perfect* weight loss diet. Pure science. The food group system is the pattern for all the healthy (and often expensive) diets in the country. Different diet programs put this pattern into different forms. Some may use columns of foods, and some may name the groups differently, or use any number of designs that conform to their image.

The food group system accomplishes many things simultaneously, and they are very important to a dieter.

- you get the protein you need for lean muscle protection – and that means better fat burn
- you get the fiber you need for fullness and better intestinal transit time – and that means less calorie absorption
- you get the 50 essential nutrients automatically – and that means health and disease prevention
- you get the calcium you need to prevent bone deterioration as you age
- you get the textures you need for chewing – and that means better appetite control
- you get pleasure from variety – it's more palatable, and less likely to make you break your diet from boredom
- you get an automatic maintenance plan – all you have to do is increase your calories across the board
- you're set for a healthy, slimmer life.

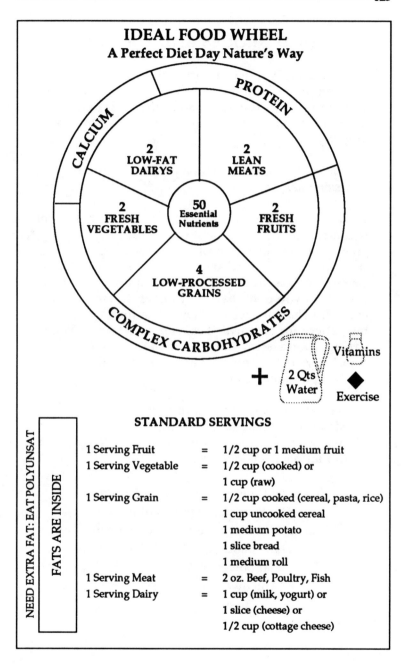

IDEAL FOOD WHEEL

A Perfect Diet Day Nature's Way

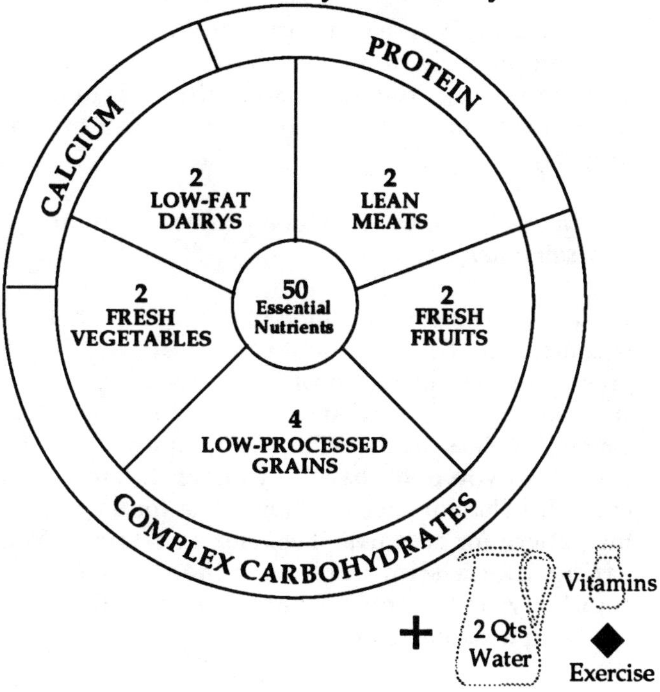

NEED EXTRA FAT: EAT POLYUNSAT

FATS ARE INSIDE

STANDARD SERVINGS

1 Serving Fruit	=	1/2 cup or 1 medium fruit
1 Serving Vegetable	=	1/2 cup (cooked) or 1 cup (raw)
1 Serving Grain	=	1/2 cup cooked (cereal, pasta, rice) 1 cup uncooked cereal 1 medium potato 1 slice bread 1 medium roll
1 Serving Meat	=	2 oz. Beef, Poultry, Fish
1 Serving Dairy	=	1 cup (milk, yogurt) or 1 slice (cheese) or 1/2 cup (cottage cheese)

FOOD GROUPS AND FAT BURN

It's simply what your metabolism needs to function properly in order to burn fat, while building and repairing tissues and cells. When your metabolism doesn't get it, it simply doesn't function properly.

The Risks: None. Anytime you use it, you're doing yourself a favor.

The Extra Benefits: Name it, it does it. Cholesterol is controlled. Sugar, fat and sodium are regulated. It gives you the nutrient profile for disease prevention. It's the diet you need to handle stress. Name something else. It does that too. An automatic habit corrector—you don't have to wonder if you're getting enough behavior modification. The food groups are the pattern for automatic behavior adjustment. You're eating like a slim person. When you follow it regularly, it becomes a habit. And it doesn't do anything negative to you.

It's nature's way to make your day.
Make your days count for something.
Just start. The magic is in real food. Straight from our farmers' laboratories.

The next time you see a field of grain
Think about the power of it
The next time you see fruit on the trees
Think about the power of it
Bring that power back into your life
You owe it to yourself
to diet right!

DAIRY ON YOUR DIET

2 Servings Daily Adults

A MUST FOR CALCIUM
AND PROTEIN

Fatter Daily Products	**Dieter's Choice Dairy**
Whole Milk Creams	2%, 1%, or skim milk buttermilk, soy milk
Yogurt Whole	Low fat yogurt plain or fruit
Eggs	Egg whites or 1 yolk to two whites
Cheeses	Skim or low fat cheeses
Cottage Cheese whole	2% cottage cheese

Do not skip your dairy products!!!!!

Limit most cheeses except dieter's choice cheeses. Cheeses are the foods that can really add on fat. Two slices of an average cheese will give you 18 grams of fat, and 54 mg of cholesterol, plus a higher level of saturated fat than unsaturated. (You want to avoid that.)

If you drink coffee or tea with cream or an imitation creamer, train yourself to drink 2% milk in your coffee or tea. Use skim for cereals.

EXTRA FATS FOR A DIETER Think about your fat cells before you add fats to your diet. They're already in your food. The rest is excess.

GRAINS ON YOUR DIET

4 Servings Daily

This is the group that often tricks dieters because they mistake processed grains, cereals, breads, and pasta mixes for the real thing. They're not. Try to find as many whole grain products as you can. Check cereals for excess sugar. Consider making your own muffins to freeze for superior whole grain boosters. It will be worth the effort when you see the fat loss and health. Whole grains have trace fat, no cholesterol, and they're the complex carbohydrates you've been missing. Remember, the grains aren't fattening, it's what you put on them. Enjoy pasta salads, potato skins with vegetables, whole wheat waffles with strawberries.

Eat any whole grain or low processed grain:

Barley
Bran
Bran flakes
Bread crumbs
Buckwheat
Bulgar
Breads, whole grain
Cornbread,muffins
Corn flakes
Cracked wheat
Crackers whole grain
Cream of wheat (not instant)
English muffins
Farina
Flour, whole wheat, soy, cornmeal
Macaroni
Millet
Muffins whole grain
Oat flakes
Oatmeal
Pancakes
Pasta
Pita
Pizza whole wheat (lite cheese)
Pizza pitas (lite cheese)
Pumpernickel
Rice wild, brown, converted yellow
Rolls, whole grain
Rye
Sesame
Shredded wheat
Spaghetti
Tortilla yellow corn
Waffles
Wheat germ
Whole wheat

MEATS, POULTRY ON YOUR DIET

Part of Protein Group
Total Protein
2 Servings Daily

Use meats in kabobs, as entrees, in stir fry, sandwiches. Use poultry in salads, casseroles, and soups. Avoid organ meats. They're super high cholesterol. Also high is turkey dark meat, cured ham, chicken (back) and frankfurters.

Poultry is lower in saturated fat than other meats. If you keep your red meat portions to 2 ounces, you can use the fatter proteins that are starred (*).

Fatter Proteins	Leaner Proteins
Bacon	Chicken white meat
Braunschweiger	Chuck roast
Bologna	Flank steak
Chicken (drum stick, thigh, wing)*	Ground beef lean
Corned beef	Ground turkey, chicken lean
Duck	Leg of lamb
Goose	Round steak
Ground beef regular	Turkey light meat
Ham	Veal cutlet
Knockwurst	Veal rib roast
Lamb chop*	Veal rump roast
Pheasant	Venison
Porterhouse steak	
Rib roast	
Rump roast*	
Sirloin steak	
T Bone steak	
Veal chuck	

SNACKS FOR A DIETER *See* Snacks.

FISH ON YOUR DIET

Part of Protein Group
Total Protein
2 Servings Daily

The standard serving size for the meat group is 2 ounces. But since fish is lighter and far less fattening than red meats, 3 ounces is acceptable for lean muscle protection. Use fish as entrees, in fish kabobs, in stir fry fares, in pita sandwiches, in fish salads. Broil or saute with an unsaturated vegetable spray, with lemon and garlic, and your favorite spices.

Lower Cholesterol Fish

Abalone
Anchovy
Bass
Bluefish
Carp
Catfish
Cod
Eel
Flounder
Frogs Legs
Haddock
Halibut
Perch Ocean
Perch Yellow
Pike
Pollock
Salmon
Sardines
Scallops
Shad
Smelt
Snails
Snapper
Trout
Wakame
Whitefish

Higher Cholesterol Fish
(Omega Oils)

Caviar
Clams
Crab
Herring
Lobster
Mackerel
Canned oysters
Shrimp
Tuna

DRINKS FOR A DIETER *See* BEVERAGES.

VEGETABLES ON YOUR DIET

2 Servings Daily Minimum

This is the best group for dieters. Versatile, pleasurable, powerful, trace fat, fabulous fiber. For salads, pasta salads, potato skin snacks, casseroles, soups, stews, entrees, sauces, snacks and low-fat dips. Name it, vegetables can do it! Eat as many vegetables fresh as you can.

Avoid garbanzo beans (fat) and use soy beans as a protein.

Eat any vegetable, legume or fresh vegetable juice:

Alfalfa sprouts
Artichoke
Asparagus
Bamboo shouts
Beans (any)
Beets
Broccoli
Brussels Sprouts
Cabbage (any)
Carrots
Carrot juice
Cauliflower
Celery
Chard
Chives
Collards
Corn
Cress
Cucumber
Dandelion
Dock
Eggplant
Endive
Garlic
Ginger root
Kale
Leeks
Lettuce (any)
Mushrooms
Mustard greens
Okra
Onions
Parsley
Parsnips
Peas
Peppers (plain & hot)
Pickles (check sodium)
Pimentos
Potato*
Pumpkin
Radish
Rutabaga
Sauerkraut
Scallions
Shallots
Spinach
Squash
Sweet potato
Tomato
Tomato juice (sugar free)
Turnips
Turnip Greens
Vegetable juice (not canned)
Water chestnuts
Watercress
Yams
Yeast (bakers, brewers)

*Potatoes baked or boiled. Avoid fried, dehydrated, hash browns, or au gratin. Potato pancakes are OK, with vegetable spray.

FRUITS ON YOUR DIET

2 Servings Daily Minimum

FRESH FRUITS OR FRESH FRUIT JUICES

One standard serving listed for fruit is 1/2 cup for dieting. But you don't have to be as rigid as that. Fruits are low in fat, good fiber sources, high-vitamin foods. Use fruits in cereals, as a topping for a whole-grain waffle or pancake, and as desserts. In water, they make great diet spritzers. When you want something sweet, have a fruit instead of candy or cake. One apple a day makes good cholesterol sense, excellent for fat loss.

OMIT THESE FRUITS: AVOCADO (FAT), DRIED FRUITS (SODIUM), FRUITS IN HEAVY SYRUP (SUGAR), GREEK OLIVES (SODIUM), COCONUT (CHOLESTEROL, PALM (CHOLESTEROL)

Eat any fruit fresh or frozen:

Acerola
Apple
Apricot
Banana
Blackberries
Blueberries
Boysenberries
Cantaloupe
Cherries
Crabapple
Cranberry
Currant
Dates
Elderberries
Figs
Fruit cocktail
Gooseberries
Grapefruit
Grapes
Guava
Kumquat
Lemon
Lime
Loganberries
Mango
Melon
Nectarine
Olives
Orange
Papaya
Peach
Pear
Persimmon
Pineapple
Plums
Pomegranate
Prickly pear
Prunes
Quince
Raisins
Raspberries
Rhubarb
Strawberries
Tangerine
Watermelon

Remember these fruit treats to spruce up meals:
Applesauce
Cranberry sauce
Apple butter

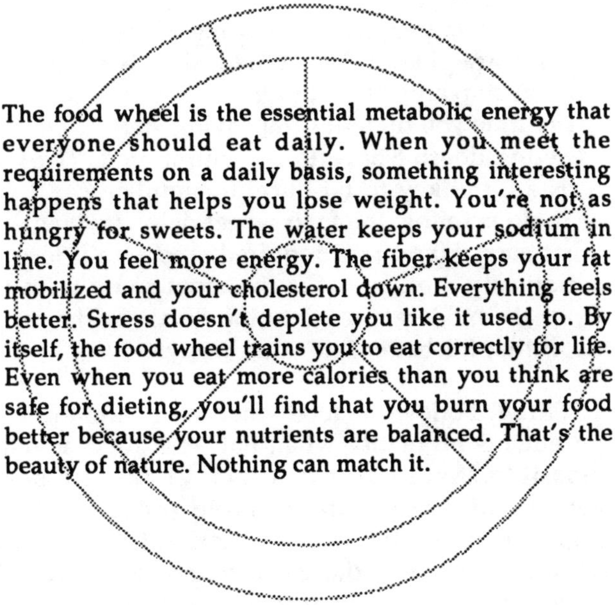

The food wheel is the essential metabolic energy that everyone should eat daily. When you meet the requirements on a daily basis, something interesting happens that helps you lose weight. You're not as hungry for sweets. The water keeps your sodium in line. You feel more energy. The fiber keeps your fat mobilized and your cholesterol down. Everything feels better. Stress doesn't deplete you like it used to. By itself, the food wheel trains you to eat correctly for life. Even when you eat more calories than you think are safe for dieting, you'll find that you burn your food better because your nutrients are balanced. That's the beauty of nature. Nothing can match it.

HOW TO DIET SUCCESSFULLY
Fix Your Day

How do you start? Do you need pre-planning, special preparations, a food scale, kit of diet mixes, special formula foods?

NO. JUST START.

Do the best you can every day!

Then, when you get in the swing of eating nature's way, do it straight out, take it to ideal body weight.

If you stop and start, it's OK.

Any time you do it, it's improving you.

Dieting doesn't have to be complicated. The food groups are the key to fat-burning simplicity. All you have to do is follow the food wheel daily, making sure you eat *everything* that's required, and you'll lose fat automatically. You can take the strict route from the start, or the moderate route to the finish, or the casual route, if that fits better into your lifestyle.

STRICT: Follow the food wheel daily and meet the requirements no matter what. Eat fresh food as much as possible. Avoid all extra fats. Cook with spray vegetable oil (unsaturated). Avoid processed foods and grains, except the whole grains that have at least the bran intact (and the germ where possible). Eat extra vegetables or fruits if you need more food, or if you are an active exerciser.

MODERATE: Follow the food wheel daily and meet the requirements no matter what. You can include extra fats, but keep an eye on them. More than 2 extra fats isn't recommended for superior fat burn. Moderate your use of processed foods, reading the labels for sugar, salt and fat content. Realize that you aren't getting the fiber you need if you eat processed foods instead of more natural foods, so you might want to tack on an apple a day to be safe. Eat fresh food whenever possible. Eat all snacks in complex carbohydrates — fruits, whole grains or vegetables. Your first job is to meet the minimum requirements on the food wheel. Consider the rest extra.

CASUAL: Diet during the weekdays and take the weekends off. However, keep an eye on your food intake on weekends, and try to moderate it. Meet the requirements on the food wheel on or off a diet. Consider the rest of your food extra and use this as a guide to finding out about your food desires and habits. Read the sections on behavior and think about adding them to your life. Practice imagery and relaxation and use this as a foundation to give you the incentive to move to the stricter plan full time for a boost in fat loss. Or you can continue with the more casual plan all the way to ideal weight.

SUPERCASUAL: Diet whenever you can, and don't feel guilty about it. The only requirement is to meet the food minimum on the daily wheel, no matter what. The rest is your decision. The important point to remember about a real food diet is that it will always benefit you because you are getting your daily nutrient needs met. Even if you do it one week every month, over time you'll start to trim down, if you don't go overboard with food on a regular basis.

NATURE'S NATURAL POWER

Eating real food is the simplest, most powerful way you can get down to ideal body weight and stay there.

You might not realize that *what you don't eat* can be as fattening as what you do eat.When you don't get your daily nutrient needs met, nothing works right, least of all weight loss.

You can eat next to nothing and fail to lose weight because you don't have your daily nutrient needs in place.You can eat more calories and still lose weight when you have your daily nutrient needs in place.

It's the secret that lean people know and follow with pleasure. They like to eat for nutrition, because of the way it makes them feel, and it automatically keeps them lean.

Obesity isn't a disease of hypernutrition, it's a disease of malnutrition. You aren't getting your daily nutrient needs met.

Obesity and overweight aren't necessarily caused by overeating. They can be caused by improper eating. You aren't getting your daily nutrient needs met.

IS THERE MAGIC IN THIS PLAN?

Dieters love magic. It's part of their dreamers' streak. Rather than let it work against you, let it work for you. Think about what you get from the food groups, when you meet your daily nutrient needs as recommended.

NATURE'S 100% ENZYME CATALYST DIET. Not just one enzyme triggered in isolation, all of them stimulated to action by the food you eat.

NATURE'S AMINO ACID BALANCE. Not one amino acid to excess, or one amino acid missing, which can hinder your protein metabolism. All of them in the proportions needed for proper metabolism.

SUCCESSFUL DIETING STYLE

If the rigid rules and standards of most American diets were successful, everyone would be thin by now. Every twenty minutes, someone is going on a diet. Often one dieter will go on and off a diet in twenty minutes. Punishment, self-denial, deprivation and restriction are adding up to weight regain. When you aren't comfortable with what you're doing, you won't keep doing it for long, and most diets are based on deprivation. That makes them something to be dreaded.

If you are a former dieter, you have to shake some old diet ghosts out of your closet. Good foods and bad foods. Guilt, blame and self-recrimination. A head war with food on a daily basis. Starving to get thin. Feeling like you're being punished because you are dieting. The list goes on and on. You know what the problems are.

Just because you are dieting, you don't have to treat yourself like you're not worth a normal life. You don't have to adopt abnormal eating patterns, eating foods you don't like and wouldn't eat unless you thought you had to.

Isn't it possible to create a world of food for yourself that will be thrilling and still be fat free? There are hundreds of foods to choose from to fashion a new world of food.

Here are some hints that might help you get started on the right track.

1. Avoid eating dry or deprived because you are dieting. There are dozens of ways to eat gourmet without cooking with fat. Tomato juice with lemon and herbs makes an excellent cooking sauce that tastes salty, but isn't. Garlic, lemon and basil make an excellent base for saute. Whole grain flours with herbs and spices make healthy gravies, with the fat skimmed off. You can stir fry with pear juice. You

can top a waffle with fresh strawberry juice. Mushrooms make a marvelous meaty gravy that is fat free. Wine vinegar and herbs add juice and flavor to meats. Ratatouille vegetables with spices make a fabulous sauce. Cocoa powder with vanilla, mixed thick with water or skim milk can be a flavored topping for desserts. Use your imagination. You don't have to cook with butter or margarine to eat fabulous.

2. What about a panic attack for something chocolate? If you've been dieting for a few weeks, or even on the first week, is something chocolate going to throw your whole system out of balance. No. Is it going to make you lose weight slower. No, not if you don't eat the whole cake. And your odds of eating a whole cake are greater if you try to deny yourself constantly, and lust after it in every window. Dieting is an art of moderation. Have a small mint patty to satisfy your chocolate urge. Or take a vanilla wafer and dot it with chocolate syrup. If you're going to hit the ceiling if you don't have a piece of chocolate cake, have a small piece, then continue with your diet the next day. Exercise regularly and you'll still be in good shape.

3. What about eating out? Should you carry a bag of *your* food and refuse to look at the menu. Should you sit there and not eat, and talk about not eating throughout the entire meal. What happens then? You go home and eat to compensate. You can eat successfully in a restaurant without feeling like an ostracized child. Choose from the leaner offerings and add side dishes of vegetables. Ask for your sauces on the side, and moderate their use. Ask the waitress to have your meal cooked without butter. Drink plenty of water and eat slowly. Don't tell

yourself you'll never be able to enjoy eating in a restaurant again, because you'll believe it. If you choose poorly this time and eat a basket of onion rings, try again the next time to eat more nutritiously. Keep up your regular eating with the food wheel as a guide and keep up your exercise. You'll make it. Believe it and you will.

4. Learn to enjoy dieting. When you eat real food, and learn to have fun in the kitchen experimenting with recipes, you get a renewed sense of food pleasure. Food pleasure is a vital part of life. A microwave diet dinner deprives you of more than fiber. It takes away the smell of food cooking, and the sensory pleasure of food. You don't have to cook with fat for that pleasure. And you don't have to dread going into the kitchen because you have excess fat. Adapt your kitchen to a leaner, healthy fare, and fill your refrigerator with healthy foods, instead of stripping it down to metal shelves with celery and cottage cheese looking lonely in there.

5. TV and Micro Dinners. Make your own variety of quick-cook dinners that you can heat up in a snap. Cook batches of soup, pasta salads, low-fat casseroles and stews, and freeze them in one meal packs. That way, you won't be caught without a healthy choice some night when you're extra hungry.

6. Learn to eat your snacks in carbohydrates, instead of sweets. Before you reach for the chocolate cream pie, eat an apple or a bowl of strawberries. Before you take the cheesecake, eat a bagel with jelly. Not only will this save you a lot of excess fat, but it will provide nutrition and satisfaction. And it is the best lean habit you can learn. Extra carbohydrates

aren't going to layer on fat. They're long chain molecules and they take a long time to digest. Many studies indicate that they never get to fat. You'd have to eat a lot of them to equal the calories and fat in one piece of cheesecake, and half way through, you'd be full.

7. Use your dieting time to learn relaxation exercises, practice meditation and read self-supportive materials that help you create a new view of life. Use positive self talk as a booster every night and morning. Learn to look at the good things that happen to you every day, and away from the bad ones. Dieting can be a resource for self-renewal that is far greater than the one note goal of weight loss. You can lose the weight you've been carrying in your mind. That makes you lighter inside, where it really counts.

IDEAL DIET WEEK

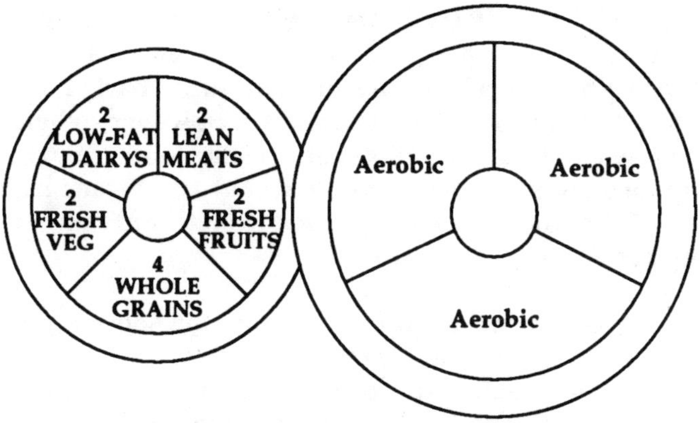

Your INPUT Drives up your OUTPUT
Your ACTIVITY Drives up your OUTPUT
RESULT: Your OUTPUT exceeds your INPUT
You burn more than you eat

Your food burns calories too from thermogenesis — the heat of eating. The wheel provides the 50 essential nutrients you need to feed your metabolism, to activate its chemical action to repair, rebuild and maintain all of your body processes, from the largest organ to the smallest cell. When you take the wheel to its low-fat format, the result is: fat burns and burns.

Your 30 minute aerobic routine, 3 x per week drives up your metabolism to burn more calories (15%+). It also builds muscle, the vital body protein you lose from poor dieting and need to rebuild, in order to be a better fat burner for life. These factors combine to revive your sluggish metabolism, align your body composition, and set you up with the status you need to stay lean after your diet.

Overall result: While fat is burning, muscle is restored. You get superior weight loss and a body composition to match. In maintenance, you will be able to raise your calorie level without regaining.

YOUR GOAL: TO GET BACK IN BALANCE

▲ **FOOD SCALE** A weight measuring device for portion control. *See* Scale (Food).

▲ **FOOD SHOPPING** Making sound diet choices. Each diet has its own shopping list for foods, and many are not foods you can find easily in your supermarket, or you have to shop in the diet sections. However, when you choose a natural food diet that uses the food groups,more options are available to you, but that also means making careful choices. It can be educational and fun, and it makes you a wise consumer.

1. Give yourself a little more time for shopping when you use the food group system for dieting. Let yourself enjoy the process, and explore the food varieties, especially in the vegetable and fruit sections.
2. Read labels on processed foods to determine which ones have the least fat, sugar, sodium and additives. Select the best possible versions of these foods (or limit them as much as possible).
3. If you shop when you're hungry, it makes sweets and bakery goods irresistible. If you find yourself getting hungry while you shop, buy an apple and eat it while you select foods. It will give you sweetness and fiber, and those urges will be dramatically decreased.
4. Make your shopping list an education system for foods by drawing it in 5 columns, headed by the food group divisions. Each time you list a food you need during the week, list it under the food group heading. You'll automatically see the group or groups you neglect. Fill in the missing groups with healthy selections and you'll be rounding out your diet regularly.
5. Buy fresh foods whenever possible, and as many whole grains as you can find.
6. Don't neglect your desserts (on the light side). When you plan these into your daily diet, you do not feel deprived or dis-satisfied. Fruit pops, frozen grapes, a

mini mint patty, angel food cake — you can allow yourself to have a dessert each day and still burn fat. That way, you won't be fooled by the candy rack that's always next to the checkout counter — it's there to grab you at the last minute. You'll be fortified with food pleasures that won't make you fat.

FOOD TRANSIT TIME The time it takes for food to pass through your intestines. Also called intestinal motility. This is a very important factor in weight gain. The longer food stays in your intestines, the more calories you can absorb and store as fat. Athletes have food transit times of 6 hours, while obese people can have food transit times as long as 24 hours. The worst thing you can do is take laxatives to speed up your food transit time, because you lose valuable minerals and nutrients. The best steps to take are to increase your fiber intake, and increase your exercise and daily activity. Both increase your food transit time. *See* Fiber. Exercise.

FORMULA DIET A program that relies on powders, drinks, or shake-and-pour supplements to replace average meals. *See* Supplements.

FORTIFIED Re-supplied with vitamins, minerals or nutrients that are lost during processing of foods, particularly grains. Standard fortification includes three B vitamins, niacin, thiamine, and riboflavin, plus iron and Vitamin C. Replacing lost vitamins and nutrients is no substitute for the original food. Fortified foods are also stripped of fiber, have added sugar, salt and fat, which the real foods don't have. If you switch to the whole grain varieties, you get ten times the nutrition at the outset. Whole grain flour beats white flour by a lean mile for cooking and gravy-making. High fiber cereals and breads made from whole grains keep your food moving through digestion and metabolism with real fat burning benefits. Many people find it difficult at first when they switch to whole grain foods, after they've been used to the smooth, sugary version of cereals and breads that go down so quickly. Re-train yourself by using half-and-half mixes. Half of the fortified kind, and half of the whole grain. Then gradually let the whole grains move the processed grains out. *See* Food Groups.

FRAME Bone structure and density. People of the same height can have different bone structure and density. This accounts for a 10 pound differential, that is not body fat. For instance, a small-framed woman of 5'4" has a recommended ideal weight of 120, while a medium-framed woman of 5'4" can weigh 130 and a large framed woman of 5'4" can weigh 140, and not be carrying excess fat. Bone weight can account for the extra pounds.

However, be careful that you don't use your frame as an excuse for extra pounds. Everyone likes to look at the height/weight tables and say: "I can weigh more because I have big bones." Then they take the highest weight on the tables and if they haven't exceeded it, they feel more comfortable about their weight. Your goal should be the *fittest* you can be, without using extreme or radical measures to achieve that fitness. That's why it's better to take the midpoint of the weight range indicated for your height, weight and frame. That way, you are setting strong, realistic goals.

➡ **How To Find Your Frame Size**

1. Extend your arm forward, palm up. Bend your forearm upward to a 90 degree angle.
2. Keep your fingers straight and turn your wrist out, away from your body.
3. Place your thumb and index finger (other hand) on the two prominent bones on each side of your elbow. Measure the space between your fingers with a ruler or tape measure.
4. Compare the measurements to the following table.

This table gives you the measurements for MEDIUM FRAMES. Anything below this measurement is a small frame, and above is a large frame.

FRAME SIZE
Based on Height in 1 Inch Heels

WOMEN		MEN	
Height	Elbow Breadth	Height	Elbow Breadth
4'10 to 4'11	2-1/4 to 2-1/2"	5'2 to 5'3	2-1/2 to 2-7/8"
5'0 to 5'3	2-1/4 to 2-1/2"	5'4 to 5'7	2-5/8 to 2-7/8"
5'4 to 5'7	2-3/8 to 2-5/8"	5'8 to 5'11	2-3/4 to 3"
5'8 to 5'11	2-3/8 to 2-5/8"	6'0 to 6'3	2-3/4 to 3-1/8"
6'0 to 6'3	2-1/2 to 2-3/4"	6'4 to 6'7	2-7/8 to 3-1/4"

FRUIT DIET A program that relies on fruits for primary calories. Or a program that uses one fruit as a magic food, such as a grapefruit after each meal. While it is true that fruits are ideal diet foods, eating fruits without eating the other food groups can lead to nutrient deficiencies, dizziness, muscle losses, and a very inferior form of weight loss. Many diets use fruits as a focus, and are called fruit diets, when in actuality, they are calorie-cutting diets that highlight fruits. Most diets look for a handle or label to separate them from other diets, and isolating fruits is one way to get that handle. The problem is, these diets have led to confusion and mis-information about foods. Many dieters learned to dislike fruits, after eating them exclusively for weeks, and feeling the effects of solo fruit diets. Eating any food to excess, without the presence of the other food groups, is unhealthy, not only because of nutrient losses in the absence of other foods, but because this kind of eating creates destructive food habits and patterns. You can start out with a fat problem and wind up with major food problems after a bout with one of these extreme food diets.

- **FRUITS** One of the essential food groups, sources of fiber, vitamins/minerals and sugar. Diet Foods. *See* Carbohydrates. Sugar.

g

GALLSTONES Hardened cholesterol/calcium deposits that are combined with bile. During digestion, your gallbladder secretes the bile needed to emulsify fats for metabolism. But bile can also be secreted by the liver. Deposits can form in the passage between your liver and gallbladder, in your gallbladder itself, or in the passage between your liver and intestines. The condition is more prevalent in people with diabetes, obesity, the elderly, and females. The recommended treatment is to avoid large meals and high fat, high cholesterol diets, and insure that you are drinking plenty of water. The condition can require surgery and should be treated by a physician.

GASTRO-INTESTINAL The parts of digestion that relate to your stomach and intestines, the two primary organs for breakdown of food into nutrients. *See* Digestion.

GENETIC The inherited tendencies for disease or health. Many diseases, including obesity, have genetic tendencies. This doesn't mean that you *will* get them. Healthy diet and exercise can minimize your risk, and even prevent many diseases from occurring. *See* Causes. Risks.

GLUCOSE The form of energy that carbohydrates take after they are digested and turned into nutrients that can be absorbed into your blood. A prime energy source for red blood cells. The simplest form of sugar. *See* Digestion.

GLUCOSE HIGH A sugar rush, usually accompanied by a dizzy feeling. It usually means your diet is too high in sugar. *See* Sugar.

GLYCOGEN The form carbohydrate nutrients take when they are stored in your body.

▲ **GOALS** Expectations. The best way to achieve your diet goal is to take one day at a time, one pound at a time using a healthy diet. This keeps you moving forward. Each step you take is an achievement, teaching you better eating and slimmer living. Over time, these habits will become natural — ingrained. This will keep you slim on a permanent basis.

GOUT Inflammation of joints caused by uric acid salt deposits in joint tissues. This is a metabolic disturbance, where excess uric acid occurs in your blood. Protein is not metabolized properly, causing salt crystals to form around fingers, toes, heels, knees or other joints. The deposits create bumps or growth that irritate your joints, and inflammation occurs. A gout attack begins in one joint and spreads to others before it abates. The pain is usually greatest in the morning, because your body processes have slowed down in sleep. An average attack can last 5-10 days or more, before abating. Reoccurrence is common. Gout is generally considered a hereditary disease that can be aggravated by obesity, aging, improper diet, overuse of alcohol, stress, and *rapid weight loss.* People with gout should avoid organ meats, since they contain purine, which can bring on an attack. The recommended treatment includes regular exercise, since that improves the circulatory system, good diet with moderate protein and low fat, and rest. The condition should be treated by a physician.

● **GRAINS** Seeds from grass such as wheat, rye, oats, rice and barley. Also called cereals, and used in flours, breads and pastas. Known as the *staff of life*. Grains can be viewed in two categories for easy reference.

WHOLE GRAINS: Grains that still contain the germ of the original grain.

HALF GRAINS: Grains that have been processed to remove the bran or germ or both. This is done to prolong the shelf life of grains, but all of the nutrients in the bran and germ are lost. These two parts are the most nutrient rich components of the grain. The half grains are then fortified or enriched to replace some of the nutrients lost in milling, but it's not the same as the real thing.

The flours used in breads are ground and sifted grains. *Whole Grain Flour* is the product of the first milling process. It contains the germ of the grain. The bran has been removed. Whole grain flours still contain many nutrients. *Bleached Flour* is refined flour, whitened to look good. Lowest in nutrients. *Enriched Flour* can be a refined flour, or all-purpose flour with added nutrients such as niacin, thiamine, riboflavin, and iron. *All Purpose Flour* is a blend of different grains, and can be mostly refined.

When you're choosing rices, the wild rices and whole grain rices are the best. But check the labels of processed rice mixes or medleys, since they can contain fat and sodium. Look for the more natural ones.

White Rice is dehulled and polished to look good. It has lost its B Vitamins but can be enriched. *Converted Rice* is the better of the white rices, slightly higher in vitamins. *Brown Rice* is a rich source of B vitamins, calcium, phosphorous and iron. *Wild Rice* is the tops! Twice the nutrients as white. *See* Food Groups.

▲ **GUILT** Self-criticism and blame. A useless emotion. *See* Relaxation to let it go.

h

▲ **HABITS** Learned behaviors that are ingrained through repetition. How is a habit formed? Usually in childhood by watching other people, or responding to situations in your own unique way. You may still use Yellow Number 9 pencils today because you used them in school during the year that you got As. Or you may not like to use blue ink because that's the ink color on report cards when you got demerits. This generation's kids will use computers instead of pens or pencils when they're adults. Some may keep computers in their bedrooms, as they're doing now. Some may start working after midnight because they're night owls now.

You can reverse a habit you had as a child because it reminds you of something that felt uncomfortable then. For instance, you always walked to school, every day, rain or shine, while your neighbor rode in a red convertible her parents gave her when she was sixteen. You don't walk anywhere now — you drive. Your car may even be red.

Your moods and attitudes can also be habits. You may wake up every morning and dread getting out of bed. There doesn't seem to be a reason for it. It's a habit you picked up somewhere along the way in life. You may get up every day at dawn and run two miles, after spending four years as a marine. You may dislike it intensely, but you do it anyway. It's a habit that was trained into you. You may eat chocolate cream pie every time you feel depressed. Somewhere along the way, you ate chocolate cream pie and it cheered you up on a bad day. It might have been yesterday that you discovered chives for the first time. Tomorrow, adding them to pasta salads or gravies instead of salt will start to become a habit.

Some habits help you gain weight, while others help you get lean. The art of behavior modification is to substitute good habits for poor ones. The more good habits you can gain to outweigh the poorer habits, the greater your chances of staying lean for life.

There are four areas to consider when you are reviewing your weight-gaining habits: Eating Habits, Exercise Habits, "Diet" – Specific Eating Habits, and Overall Daily Habits. As you can see, these add up to the habits that make your lifestyle, or whole day. To see real results, you shouldn't expect to change all of these habits AT THE SAME TIME. That's too much change to introduce into your life at one time, and change causes stress. The best way to make positive habit changes is to change one or two at a time, practicing the new habit until you do it naturally, on automatic pilot. Then you can change other habits in the same way. Slow, steady change is the best way to make a new habit last. If you try to shake up your whole life overnight for a diet, before long, you'll be back to your old habits again.

➠ How to Change Weight-Gaining Habits

EATING Habits

CHANGE YOUR NO-FOOD PLAN TO A REGULAR FOOD PLAN THAT INSURES YOUR DAILY NUTRITION.

This is the first, best habit to change. Where do you get a regular food plan that is easy to start? *See* Food Groups.

EXERCISE HABITS
CHANGE YOUR NO-ACTION PLAN TO A REGULAR ACTION PLAN. 3 x PER WEEK, AEROBIC, 30 MINUTES A SESSION.
How do you choose which exercise to do? *See* Exercise.

DIET-RELATED HABITS
USE SKILLPOWER INSTEAD OF WILLPOWER TO GET TO IDEAL WEIGHT
How do you become a skillfull dieter? *See* all Behavior Keys ▲ for a state-of-the art plan.

DAILY HABITS
CHANGE NO PRIORITY SETTING TO REGULAR PRIORITY REVIEW.
How do you set priorities? *See* Lifestyle. And Behavior Keys ▲, Specifically Stress.

❤ **HDL** High Density Lipoprotein. Good Cholesterol in your body. *See* Cholesterol.

HEALTH A state of well-being that is free of disease, and usually low-risk or risk-free for the major lifestyle diseases, such as hypertension, heart disease, diabetes and cancer. This implies many things. First, that you are at your ideal body weight, and that you got there in a healthy way. Second, you don't use addictive substances or sleeping aids. It also means that you adhere to the basic dietary guidelines for good health. To be considered healthy, you also have to use exercise on a regular basis. Most of the conditions of ill-health can be dramatically improved by a healthy diet for weight loss, since that automatically includes the factors needed for overall health. But is that all there is to health? It must include a good attitude, sense of purpose, stress control, self-respect and even, spiritual beliefs. The definition of health is an issue that can go on indefinitely, since health itself is never static, At any given moment, old cells are dying in your body while new ones are being created. At the same time, the environment is changing, creating new situations that will affect health.

In addition, you can have diabetes that is being controlled, and you can still be very healthy. The key to health,more than anything, is found in the efforts you make to achieve it. Seeking positive things, and continuing to seek the positive, is the foundation of a healthy life.

When it comes to weight loss, most people don't realize that the *process* is far more important than a weight goal on the scale. When the process is positive, the results are positive, and the weight goal becomes secondary to the thrill of health. When you diet healthy, everything else takes care of itself. This year, resolve to diet healthy. It's the best thing you can do for your life.

HEALTH BENEFITS, OF EXERCISE *See* Exercise.

HEALTH RISKS Weight-related diseases or disorders. *See* Risks.

HEIGHT/WEIGHT TABLES Averages of people by weight and height, in relation to mortality statistics.

Height/weight tables are accurate indicators of height, but vague indicators of ideal body weight. The weights do not reflect body composition, simply overall weight. That's like weighing a one gallon container of water that is sealed, guessing that it's primarily water inside. The weight could be sugar and water, or it could be part water and part fat. In the case of your body, it has fat, muscle and water. Your fat content is important, but your muscle content is far more important, because that determines how much fat you can keep gaining. The water content should remain stable at all times for proper metabolism and health, and water is 55-60% of your overall weight.

Dieters spend so much energy reading their weights on scales, unaware that those 5 pound up and downs can be water fluctuations, not fat loss or gain. A major part of the weight loss seen in the first week or two on a rapid weight loss diet is water, but you think you're losing fat because the scale says five pounds less. When you see your weight as a general indicator, and your body composition as the key to better weight loss, you'll be making a major step forward to ideal body weight in the right proportions.

Body weight is a personal and sensitive issue. Numbers on weight tables should never be read as judgments or rating systems for your sense of self-worth. They are simply numbers for ideal goals. You can be ideal at a higher weight, if you're comfortable there and it isn't a weight-risk issue. Or you can go for the gold in fitness, which is reaching your desirable weight with a higher content of body muscle, just for the thrill of health and maintenance. If you change your scale-reading habit to a label-reading habit to get the weight out of your food, you'll reach the numbers on weight tables with a body composition to match. *See* Ideal Weight for the height/weight tables. *See* Scale to find the facts about your body composition, which is a better measure of fitness than *weight* alone.

● **HERBS & SPICES** Salt replacers, seasonings, and taste enhancers for dieters. Herbs and spices provide taste and pleasure, in addition to nutrition. You can use them in sauces and gravies to replace salt, fat and sugar, without feeling deprived. They make excellent teas, and garnishes for salads, soups, casseroles, stews. They can spice up potato skins for low-fat snacks. Set up an herb and spice rack in your kitchen to take the place of all the salty condiments that lead to sodium excess, and eventually hypertension. Don't confuse the real herbs and spices with the herb or spice SALTS that are available in your supermarket. The salts contain sodium or MSG.

Choose the POWDER versions, but it might help to glance at the labels to be sure. There are a variety of spices to choose from. The fresher the better.

Basil	Curry	Paprika
Bay Leaf	Dill	Parsley
Caraway	Fennel	Peppers
Celery Seed	Garlic	Poppy Seeds
Chervil	Ginger	Pumpkin Spice
Chili Powder	Marjoram	Rosemary
Cinnamon	Mustard	Saffron
Cloves	Nutmeg	Sage
Coriander	Onion	Tarragon
Cumin	Oregano	Thyme

HORMONE A chemical produced in one organ for a specific use in another organ during metabolism.

HUNGER, PHYSIOLOGICAL The need for nutrients. Biological hunger. It is controlled by your appetite center. *See* Appetite.

▲ **HUNGER, PSYCHOLOGICAL** Desire for food (as opposed to a *need* for food.) Sometimes called "imaginary hunger," or conditioned hunger.
Hunger that follows feelings – such as anxiety, depression, boredom, fear, confusion.
Hunger based on habit – repeating a pattern of eating that was learned in the past, such as eating to ease stress. You can have a conditioned response to eat certain foods for reward, such as chocolate, ice cream, sweets. Often these foods were used for rewards in childhood, or withheld for punishment.
Hunger from food cues – such as seeing food, smelling food, or being in the presence of food. You can respond to the sight of food with an increase in salivation and blood

insulin levels, as in biological hunger.

Psychological hunger is real, because you feel it, but it is not triggered by your body's need for nutrition, it is cued from a learning process. It's similar to an actor in a play, being *cued* to recite his lines after certain music, action, or gestures – and after constant rehearsals – except you are cued to eat. Eating will not satisfy the real need for emotional comfort, and in most cases, eating will only increase the problems, creating guilt and feelings of helplessness after the eating is over. Something is needed instead of food. That's where behavior modification comes in. Using behavior skills, you learn to recognize your non-biological hunger, and deal with it. Once you identify the cues, habits and moods that lead you to eat, you use your knowledge to change your responses and routines. In this sense, hunger becomes a catalyst to use for self-improvement.

HYDROGENATED A process used to turn a vegetable oil fat into a harder fat, so it will be solid at room temperature for use as a spread. *See* Cholesterol.

HYPERPLASTIC Fat cells that are normal-sized, but occur in greater numbers. Common to adolescent-onset obesity. *See* Fat Cells.

HYPERTHYROIDISM Hormone overproduction by your thyroid. Excessive thyroid hormones speed up your body processes, particularly your metabolism. This causes your nutrients to be used at a faster rate. The symptoms are sudden weight loss, rapid pulse, nervousness, fatigue, weakness, goiter. Since nutrient depletion can be extreme, muscle losses occur with hyperthyroidism. The recommended treatment is an increased nutrient diet with extra protein for muscle losses, and vitamin B complex for metabolism of extra protein and carbohydrates. This condition should be treated by a physician.

HYPERTROPHIC Fat cells swollen with fat. Common to adult-onset obesity. *See* Fat Cells.

HYPOGLYCEMIA Low blood glucose, brought about by overproduction of insulin, which removes glucose from the blood. Hypoglycemia can be caused by several factors. Eating too much refined sugar can cause your blood sugar to rise rapidly. This, in turn prompts your pancreas to secrete insulin. When too much insulin circulates regularly, too much glucose is removed. Underlying disorders can lead to hypoglycemia also, such as tumors in your pancreas that stimulate overproduction of insulin, or it can be caused by liver disorders. The symptoms are fatigue, constant hunger, weak legs, swollen feet, tight chest, headaches, eyeaches, pain, nervousness, insomnia, and often mental disorders. Reducing the consumption of refined sugars in your diet guards against the disease. A glucose tolerance test is recommended. The disease should be treated by a physician.

HYPOTHYROIDISM Hormone underproduction by your thyroid. This is generally caused by heredity, and includes an iron deficiency. Symptoms are decreased appetite, fatigue, insomnia, dry skin and hair, constipation. This condition should be treated by a physician.

IDEAL BODY WEIGHT The recommended weight for your height, sex, and frame, that gives you the best disease-prevention status. These weights assume that you have a high-muscle, low-fat body at your ideal (See Scale for body fat ratings.) If you are small-framed, you should weigh less than these values at ideal. If you are large framed, you can weigh more.

WOMEN			MEN		
Height FT	IN	Weight	Height FT	IN	Weight
4	10	96-107	5	2	118-129
4	11	98-110	5	3	121-133
5	0	101-113	5	4	124-136
5	1	104-116	5	5	127-139
5	2	107-119	5	6	130-143
5	3	110-122	5	7	134-147
5	4	113-126	5	8	138-152
5	5	116-130	5	9	142-156
5	6	120-135	5	10	146-160
5	7	124-139	5	11	150-165
5	8	128-143	6	0	154-170
5	9	132-147	6	1	158-175
5	10	136-151	6	2	162-180
5	11	140-155	6	3	167-185
6	0	144-159	6	4	172-190

Small Framed Women Can Weigh 4-6 Pounds Less Than The Lowest Number. Large Framed Women Can Weigh 10-12 Pounds More Than The Highest Number.

Small Framed Men Can Weigh 6-8 Pounds Less Than The Lowest Number. Large Framed Men Can Weigh 12-14 Pounds More Than The Highest Number.

These tables are based on lean versions of the Metropolitan Life Tables, which allowed too much weight in recent years.

▲ **IMAGERY** The skill to imagine or visualize yourself successful with future goals. *Seeing* yourself slim and healthy. *Picturing* yourself successful. Imagery exercises are used in weight control to strengthen your mind's ability to claim or own what you want (a slimmer, healthy body), so that it will become more attainable and feel more real when you achieve it.

Imagery exercises are especially helpful if you have always been overweight, since the thinner image at the end of a diet can seem unrealistic or out of reach, because you've never felt it, never experienced it firsthand. The exercises allow you to experience the feelings of being slim, even when you are currently overweight. This lifts a great weight off your internal belief systems that keep repeating that you are fat and keep you feeling fat. Combine the power of imagery with a healthy fat burning diet, and the weight can be lifted off for life.

➡ **How To Do Thin-Within Imagery**

The first step to thin-within imagery is to get a clear picture of yourself as a slimmer, healthy person. To do this, sit in a comfortable chair and let your entire body relax. (Close your eyes.) Let go of all distractions. Bring the picture into your mind of a slimmer you. Once you get your picture, let yourself experience what it feels like to be the slim you. Can you feel your muscles, and a new sense of your body? Let yourself feel the movements of slim you. Are they graceful, strong, confident? Feel the climate and the clothes you are wearing. Locate yourself in pleasant surroundings, feel the air on your skin. Feel yourself walking, running, swimming, playing tennis with friends. Feel yourself breathing in and out. Now bring the image into the present and believe that you exist this way NOW. Talk to yourself, saying: " I feel strong and happy," or describing what *you* feel. Always use the present tense, such as "I am...," not "I will be...." This is NOW. You are slim and healthy. Suspend all doubt that enters your mind, forget your present weight, and believe you are slim NOW. Let yourself feel this way for a few minutes, then open your eyes and go on with your day.

Try to use this technique 3 times each day for 5 minutes when you wake in the morning, once in midday, and again before retiring in the evening. It's a powerful, exhilarating feeling to let go of your weight. *See* Visualization.

INCHES Weight loss measurements that are usually preferred to pounds on scales, since they don't fluctuate as regularly.

INNER SELF The unique collection of attributes that make you distinct and different from everyone else. The inner self is often called the *real self* because it is not subject to superficial views of self-worth and self-value, such as appearance, physique, weight, or social opinions of worth such as money, clothes, popularity, or position in society. The inner self isn't rewarded by these things. It is rewarded by *feelings* of wellbeing and self-value, and often that means having spiritual beliefs as the source of strength. The inner self is the most valuable factor in weight loss, because you can change your outer self (get thinner), but still not satisfy your inner self.

● **INPUT** Calories eaten, specifically on a daily basis. Input is one half of the energy scale that determines your weight, or weight regulation. The balanced state is:

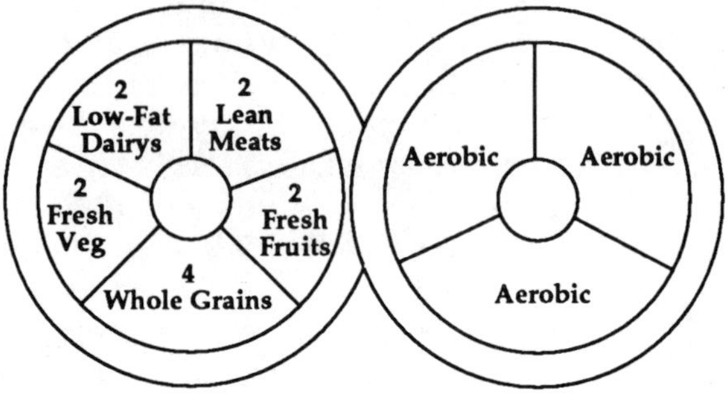

Input Equals Output
Calories Eaten Equal Calories Burned

Imbalances exist in the energy scale in overweight and the dieting phase. *See* Obesity, for the total picture.

INSULIN A hormone produced by your pancreas to help metabolize glucose—the nutrient derived from carbohydrates in digestion. After a meal, insulin is secreted. This causes your system to go into a nutrient storage phase, to save part of the nutrients from digestion. Your liver stores glucose as glycogen, your adipose tissue stores fatty acids as lipids. Other nutrients from digestion were absorbed and are circulating in your blood. These nutrients are delivered to the cells for energy for metabolism. A few hours after your meal, when the blood supply of nutrients is depleted, insulin decreases and your pancreas secretes another hormone—glucagon. This causes nutrients to be released from storage for use as energy. Your liver releases stored glucose, your adipose tissue releases fatty acids, and metabolism continues, this time from stored nutrients. This process is repeated with each meal. It's your body's way of conserving and metering out nutrients so that it can maintain itself throughout the day.

In diabetes, not enough insulin is produced, or none is produced. The process for metabolizing carbohydrates is not possible, and glucose metabolism is inhibited. *See* Diabetes Type I.

◆ **INTERVAL TRAINING** A method for gradually developing your aerobic potential without stress or strain. Interval training is a fail-safe way for beginners to build their fitness levels gradually. It lets you start at your own pace and gradually increase your speed and build endurance. You use timed bouts of exercise and follow with rest periods to enable you to last the full exercise session. This is especially important for beginners on exercise machines.

Your exercise sessions start off with short bouts and gradually increase in duration, according to your progress. The exercise bouts are continued until they total 20 to 30 minutes of aerobic activity. Beginning exercisers finish with the satisfaction of knowing they completed the same workout a seasoned exerciser would, but without jeopardizing their health or motivation.

How To Do Interval Training

- Start with 3 — 5 minutes on a machine at a slow pace, or as your target heart rate dictates.
- Take 2 — 4 minutes off, but keep moving — walk around the room until your heart rate slows down.
- *Never stop completely!* This would shock your system.
- Do another 3 - to 5-minute session, then stop and walk around.
- Complete 6 sessions.

As your fitness level improves, the length of each session can be increased, but continue to monitor your heart rate. Do not wait until you get symptoms of overexertion such as dizziness or nausea — these are danger signals.

Good ventilation is critical. Work out in areas with good air flow. If necessary, set up a fan. Given the oxygen demands of this high-intensity aerobic activity, make sure that you have plenty of ventilation and wear cool clothing that breathes. Evaporation of sweat is what keeps your internal body temperature regulated.

Remember: You are not in competition with anyone but yourself. There are varying levels of fitness that can be attained. Use your target heart rate as a guide to increasing the duration of your exercise session. Just the thrill of feeling and seeing yourself improve is worth every ounce of sweat.

You should strive to increase the length of your exercise session every 2 — 4 weeks, but you will need to be faithful to your workout routine in order to attain this goal. This pace of advancement is not mandatory. Go at your own pace. An interval workout is the same as one long exercise sessions. *See* Exercise.

INTESTINAL MOTILITY The speed at which your intestines digest and eliminate food. *See* Food Transit Time. Digestion.

◆ **ISOMETRICS** An exercise technique based on tensing muscles, holding the tension, then relaxing, often against a stationary object. Muscle resistance. It can be used to tone specific areas and is good for toning the skeletal muscles.

j

◆ **JOGGING** An aerobic exercise.

Benefits:
- Excellent cardiovascular training.
- Excellent calorie-burning activity.
- Convenient: requires only the time to get dressed, warm up, and go.
- Able to enjoy the fresh outdoors, altering your path for variety.
- Easily transferred to an indoor track.
- High degree of peer support.

Guidelines:
- Jogging should not be an exercise choice if you are more than 30 pounds over your goal weight.
- A walk-jog pattern can be incorporated (walk 5 minutes, jog 2 minutes, for example) as you gradually improve your level of fitness.
- Make sure you have very supportive running shoes and proper attire for the climate.
- Stop jogging (and walk) if you experience side cramps or any muscle or joint pains.
- Always warm up with stretching to avoid injury.

Some bodies are better structured for jogging then others. Yet, with any body type, there's a high risk of injury to knees, ankles, and calves because of pounding on hard surfaces.

- **JUNK FOOD** A subjective view of food. To some people junk foods are empty calorie foods such as cola, jelly beans, taffy — 100% sugar. To others, junk foods are ones with little nutrient value for the calories, such as refined and processed foods, vending machine foods, cinema snacks, candy. Many processed foods contain all of the requirements for junk foods — high sodium, high sugar, high fat, few vitamins and minerals, lots of additives, minimal fiber. To certain age groups, junk foods are preferred foods, such as burgers, fries, chips, franks and shakes. To vegetarians, junk foods can be meats. To kids who don't like to eat spinach, that can be a junk food. To Popeye, it would be a power food.

The point is, seeing food as junk, regardless of the food, isn't good food sense. In areas of the world where there is no food, jelly beans would seem like manna, and they would provide a form of energy, even if it isn't the best. Extreme attitudes about food aren't healthy, because they can create food fears in your mind. When you tell yourself, "I can't have that," your first instinct is to want it. When you say "I can have it, but I don't want it," you're gaining control over food, instead of food controlling you.

The best way to handle your versions of "junk" foods is to learn the ingredients and make sensible decisions about those foods and you.

Ask yourself: How much nutrition am I getting for the calories? Does it replace other foods in my diet? Many people rely on low-nutrition foods for bursts of sugar energy, and they never get real nutrition on a daily basis.

The best plan for a dieter is to aim for the most nutritionally-dense foods during the weight loss phase to get the best fat burn. Later, in maintenance, you can reevaluate your "junk" foods, and see if they fit into your diet in a more restricted way, one that you can handle without gaining weight. Of course, by then, you may not want low nutrition foods anymore. Somehow, they lose their magic when you realize what's in them, and the price you paid in weight gain.

How To Find The Low Nutrition Foods

HIGH SUGAR FOODS. The foods that have large quantities of excess sugar are not the best for you. These include colas, many sodas, and fruit drinks, since they contain 10-12 teaspoons of sugar in each can and provide empty calories.

HIGH SUGAR/FAT FOODS. Usually the high sugar foods are also high in fat, and it may be the *fat* that makes the sugar food so palatable. Check the labels on cereals to see if they are high in sugar and have added fats. Some cereals can have 2-4 teaspoons of sugar in 1 cup. Sweets and desserts are high sugar and high fat foods that provide little real nutrition because they are often over-processed. Cakes, pies and ice cream fit in this category. That doesn't mean that you should never eat a slice of pie again. Select the ones with less sugar and fat, and if you make pies or cakes at home, modify your recipes to be less fattening. While you are dieting, it's best to avoid these foods, or learn to moderate your use of them by eating smaller portions less often. A piece of cake once a week will not add on a pound of fat, but cake every night will add up fast. Chocolate bars and candy bars provide a few carbohydrates, but the sugar and fat they contain are not worth the risk. If you rely on candy for quick boosts of energy, switch to fruit or grains instead.

HIGH SODIUM FOODS. You can find foods that are low in sugar and fat, but high in sodium, which is bad for your heart and overall health. Many canned foods are high sodium, so check the labels. Also be sure you're not adding extra sodium in cooking and at the table.

You will find that limiting sugar, fat, and sodium in your diet is the automatic way to lose your extra weight. Often, you can make the greatest impact on your diet by simply limiting the high-sugar foods, since they usually have those hidden fats that add so much weight.

If you have a particular food you eat to excess, and it's one that is not nutritious, slowly train yourself away from that food by cutting your portions in half, then to one-fourth, then to one-eighth. Also eat it less frequently, and slowly decrease the frequency from eating it every day, to every other day, to once a week, then once a month. This is the best way to re-train yourself to *not need* this food.

k

KETOGENIC DIETS Diets that produce excess ketones from carbohydrate restriction. Some experts feel that ketone-producing diets should be avoided, since they are associated with muscle tissue wasting. Others claim there is use for these diets in cases of severe or morbid obesity, where the overweight condition is life-threatening. It is believed that muscle losses are acceptable in very obese people, since they have more muscle tissue, along with excess fat tissue. In these cases, measuring ketones with the use of a ketostick is seen as an aid in compliance, since dieters can see if they are adhering to the program by measuring their ketone output in daily urine. However, this is a subject of continued debate among scientists, since the risk/benefits ratio is unclear. KETONE DIETS CANNOT BE USED BY PEOPLE WITH INSULIN DEPENDENT TYPE I DIABETES. ALSO, KETONE DIETS SHOULD NOT BE USED WITHOUT MEDICAL SUPERVISION.

If you are *not* in your doctor's care for your diet, a ketone-producing diet is not a good choice. The primary source of energy for your muscles is *glucose from carbohydrates.* This is your body's and brain *preferred* energy. If you have no carbohydrate energy in your body, your muscles can use ketones for metabolism, and your brain can use ketones, but this is a situation that is also associated with famine conditions. The best form of fat burn occurs with balanced diets that are high in carbohydrates, and you don't suffer muscle losses. Even if you are obese, this is the best way to burn fat and protect yourself against weight regain at maintenance.

KETONES Byproducts of fat metabolism, specifically in low-or no carbohydrate diets. Ketones are sometimes called incompletely burned fat. They are also produced during anaerobic exercise, when oxygen supply is limited. *See* Exercise, Anaerobic.

KETOSIS A metabolic state usually associated with no- or low carbohydrate diets, where ketones are produced as byproducts of weight loss.

KILOGRAM A weight measurement that equals 2.2 pounds.

▲ **KITCHEN** A food cue. An environment that inspires you to eat.

There are two schools of thought about kitchen problems for dieters, and the diet you choose will dictate what skill you should use — either Approach, or Avoidance.

The problem with diets that are too different from everyday life is that they have no relationship to your real food issues. Therefore, they can't really solve them. And the feeling of being ostracized is associated with dieting, and that makes dieting seem like a negative thing. At their best, they can help you lose weight, but you've got to go through the entire Approach phase to re-learn how to relate to your real life. It's a lot to expect from a person with a weight/food problem. It drags out the diet process, and makes the whole business take so long.

Avoidance	Approach
Rationale: Since food cues make you eat, the best course is to minimize the food cues, stay away from food.	**Rationale:** Since you have to deal with food, and the problem isn't going to go away, learn how to take charge of it.
Theme: DON'T DEAL WITH FOOD DECISIONS WHILE ON A DIET. USE A FOLLOW-ALONG PLAN. SAVE FOOD DECISIONS FOR MAINTENANCE	**Theme:** DEAL WITH FOOD DECISIONS WHILE YOU'RE ON A DIET, AND FOOD PROBLEMS WILL BE SOLVED BY THE TIME YOU REACH MAINTENANCE.
Flaw: By maintenance, it's too late. You haven't learned the skills you need to avoid weight regain. Food still has all those old associations.	**Advantage:** You carry over the skills you learned, and adapt them to a higher calorie level. Food doesn't threaten you like it did. Weight regain is less likely.
Where it's most commonly used: In diets that are different from normal eating plans, such as diets with food replacement supplements, special foods, or eating styles that are not average.	**Where it's most commonly used:** In diets that are similar to normal eating plans, but are lower in overall calories, and based on nutrient density of foods.
Common avoidance techniques: Strip the kitchen of all non-diet foods.	**Common approach techniques:** Learn what's in the food you're eating so you can choose wisely.
Eat only certain foods.	Eat less fats and more carbohydrates. Moderate your food intake.
If you have a family, keep your food separate from their food.	If you have a family, your food isn't different from their food, you just eat better.

The advantage to diets that are natural and lifestyle-related is that they are patterns for how to eat healthy and still lose weight. They don't disrupt your lifestyle, and they don't create a gap between dieting and maintaining. As a result, you are less likely to fall into the gap when you come off your diet and start maintaining your new weight. And they make kitchens places where you can feel safe. *See* Cooking.

1

▲ **LABEL READING** Food education made easy. Reading the labels on foods in the supermarket is a sure-fire way to wake you up quickly to the sources of your fat, sugar and salt problems. First read the sections on sugar, sodium and additives to get the information you need for expert label reading. Then take a day and investigate the labels of the most common foods you eat. Food is the fuel for your metabolism and the source of your health and energy. One day in the supermarket can make your future lean.

How To Read Labels

Foods are listed on labels *in order of their weight* in the product. If you pick up a cereal and sugar is listed first, that means sugar outweighs all the other ingredients in the box. You're eating sugar, not a grain product. You can pick up a pack of granola bars, a substitute for candy, isn't that right? Sugar can be the first ingredient on the label. You can pick up a cereal that has sugar listed first, grains listed about mid-point, and ten different additives — and the product is called a Natural Wheat Cereal, meaning that the wheat part, which is minimal by weight, is a natural wheat. What are you going to do? Pick the best products with the least fat, sugar, salt and additives. Then make sure you fill in your diet with fresh vegetables for fiber that will be missing from these processed foods.

Label Guide To Diet Foods:

Read the labels on diet foods, using the same technique as above. Diet foods are divided into three basic categories:

1. Light or Lite. The food inside contains no more than 40 calories per ounce. The food must be similar in taste, smell and texture to the food it is representing, but it must contain at least 1/3 less calories than an equal quantity of that food.
2. Low Calorie. The food inside contains no more than 40 calories per ounce. As to what makes up those calories, you have to check the sugar and fat content.
3. Reduced Calories. The food inside must contain at least 1/3 less calories than an equal quantity of the same food. You have to check the fat and sugar calories.

At first you might feel defeated when you start reading the labels on foods in your supermarket. But don't give up. After you discover what's really in the foods you're eating, and what is not, you'll be surprised how quickly you pick up on the food game in packaging and advertising. The choices you make will automatically become better ones. Each choice is a big step toward better nutrition and fat burn. It will not only make you a better dieter, it's food education you can use for life.

The Label Game

The importance of label reading cannot be stressed too much. Think about a cola. Then think about taking the ingredients listed on a label and making a cola of your own, just to see what you're getting. Take 10 teaspoons of sugar and put it in a glass. Add a touch of coloring. Take a teaspoon of salt (to represent all the additives) spray it with food coloring and add it to the glass. Add water, shake and add ice. Makes you think twice about refreshment, doesn't it?

You can do this with an assortment of your favorite fattening foods. Be creative and show your friends. It will de-fat you. Take a piece of cake (find your favorite on the supermarket shelf and read the label). Go home and make a mix of white flour, sugar, liquid bacon fat, and salt to represent the additives. Think about baking it.

Labels can teach you everything you need to know about food. It's the quickest way to help you reduce the excesses in your diet. You don't have to cut these foods out forever. Limit them. Ration them. Put them in their proper place. Make a game out of them. When you don't buy them, the manufacturer's snap into action, and start producing better varieties. So everybody wins.

LACTOSE Sugar in dairy products, naturally occurring. Or refined and added to other foods. *See* Sugar.

LBM Lean body mass. Also called body muscle, body protein, or muscle tissue. Lean body mass is usually a combination of muscle weight, water weight and bones. It is generally assumed that everything that IS NOT FAT is your lean body mass, or fat-free mass. *See* Weight.

LDL Low Density Lipoprotein. Bad Cholesterol in your body. *See* Cholesterol.

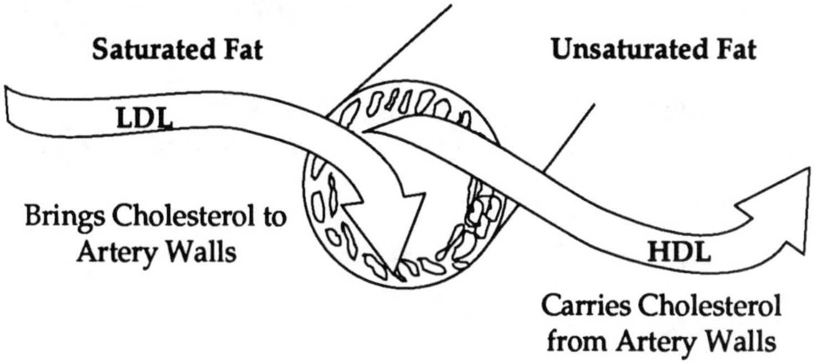

▲ **LIFESTYLE** A series of habits that make your day. A single habit is a behavior that is learned and ingrained by repetition. For instance, what's the first thing you do in the morning when you get out of bed? Brush your teeth? Do a few stretching exercises? Head for the coffee pot? These are habits. How do you eat breakfast? At the table? On the run? In the car? None? Habits. How do you handle stress? Get angry? Take a tranquilizer? Eat? Habits.

Your lifestyle is the sum of habits you do each day from the time you wake to the time you reset the alarm at bedtime. Even your sleeping patterns fall into the lifestyle picture. Step by step, from morning to night, your habits create a pattern of life (your style) that can be healthy or harmful, that can add or subtract weight.

To create a lifestyle that leads to ideal weight and health, you need more than a food restricted diet. You need to take conscious charge of your habits.

To do this, you need to know the patterns of your normal lifestyle and what you can do to make it work for you instead of against you.

The quickest way to get a complete picture of your lifestyle is to make a Lifestyle Pie. This is a behavior modification skill to make you aware of your current habits.

➡ **How To Make A Lifestyle Pie**

Use the *Lifestyle Pie* design on the opposite page.

Fill in everything you do in one day as you do it, and include the time. Use the bottom of the page to make notes about your reactions to particular issues, your feelings, or comments you want to make. Use the back side of the page if you need more room.

Make a Pie for at least 4 days including 2 weekend days, to get an accurate picture of your lifestyle.

Review your Lifestyle at the the end of each day.

MAKE A FEW COPIES OF OUR LIFESTYLE PIE

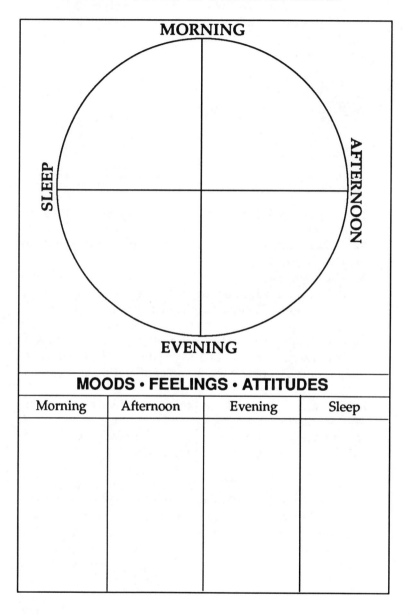

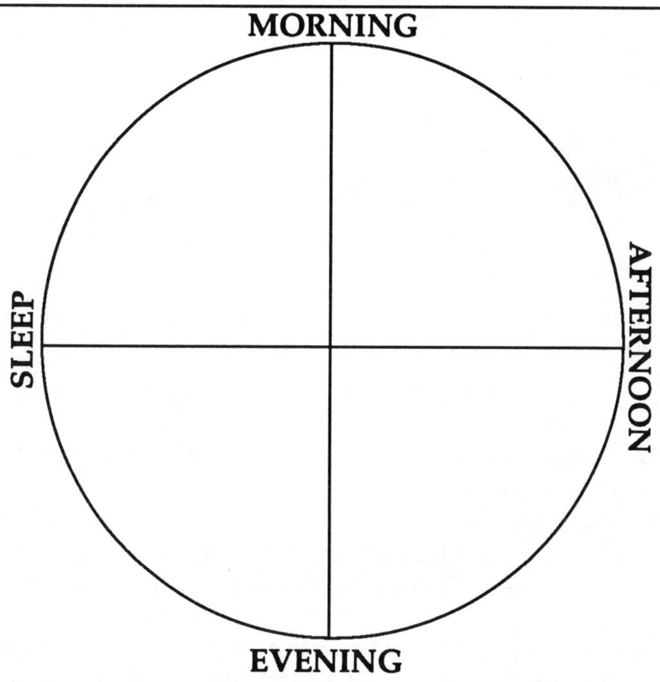

MOODS • FEELINGS • ATTITUDES

Morning	Afternoon	Evening	Sleep

● Food Skills ▲ Behavior Skills ◆ Exercise Skills

How To Create A Slim Lifestyle

What kind of lifestyle do you need to get lean and stay lean? You need to add the following slices as a routine part of your week.

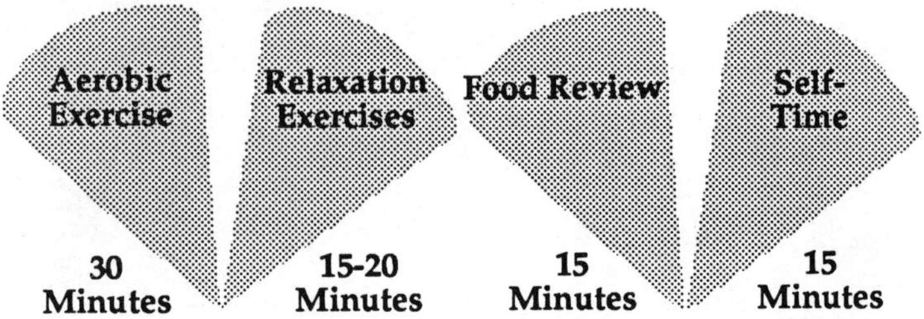

1. Aerobic exercise every *other* day for 30 minutes. *See* Exercise.
2. Relaxation exercises every day. *See* Relaxation. Meditation. Breathing.
3. Food Review Daily. *See* Food Groups.
4. Self-Time Daily. For any self-strengthening exercise. *See* Imagery. Positive Self Talk. Behavior Topics ▲.

If you use this plan during your diet, you will reach ideal weight in the best physical and emotional shape to maintain your weight. The new you that emerges at the end of your diet phase will be an exhilarating experience.

LIFESTYLE CHECKUP. Make a new Lifestyle Pie every four weeks to see how you are improving, or if you are falling back into old habits and patterns that lead to weight gain. Adjust your Pie regularly.

ADVANCED LIFESTYLE PIE. Once you've added your slices of life to your Pie, and are comfortable with them, you can move on to advanced lifestyle study. Look at your other habits and see which ones need changing. The new strength you've gained from healthy eating, regular exercise, and positive self-support will give you confidence to achieve other goals. *See* Habits.

▲ **LIFESTYLE CHANGE** Substituting healthy habits for unhealthy ones, in order to improve your style of life. If you see your lifestyle as a chain of habits that link together to make your day, then each habit is a link in the chain. When one link is weak, the chain is weakened. If three or four links are weak, the chain can break. To change your lifestyle, you take one habit at a time and strengthen it. Since the chain is interconnected, when you strengthen the weak links, you are strengthening the whole chain. The weakest links for dieters are exercise, food, and self-empowering techniques such as relaxation, meditation, and positive reinforcement on a regular basis. When you strengthen these four links, you can reach ideal weight and maintain it. *See* Lifestyle, to find out how to do it.

▲ **LIFESTYLE DIET** A program that uses exercise and behavior modification as part of its healthy diet program. The key here is healthy diet, because a program can use behavior modification and exercise, but the diet might not be up to par. A healthy diet is one that uses all the food groups in a lower calorie setting, so that you get all your essential nutrients and learn how to use food to accomplish your fitness goals. That way, you're set for life, because you can deal with real food in the real world where the problems began. When you settle for less in a diet, everybody wins but you. Learn to expect more from a diet than weight loss that doesn't last. You're worth it. And your body will thank you for it. You'll see the difference in health, wellbeing and weight maintenance. *See* Food Groups.

LIPIDS Fat deposits in your cells or blood. Also called triglycerides.

LIPOPROTEIN A substance in your body that contains fat (lipid) and protein. It's the substance that carries cholesterol in your blood. *See* Cholesterol.

LIPOSUCTION Surgery to remove fat cells. *See* Fat Cells.

LIQUID PROTEIN DIETS Diets that were blamed for deaths from chronic muscle losses. These diets were a fad more than a decade ago, and consisted of liquid drinks which were high protein. It was found that the form of protein used in these formulas was a non-metabolic variety, and this caused loss of muscle from vital organs such as the heart. Your body needs protein to rebuild its cells and muscle, including protein for hemoglobin in your blood. It must get the protein in the form of amino acids in the pattern needed to make a new protein. Eight of the amino acids can't be made by your body, and you must get them from food. The protein in these liquid diets did not provide the amino acids that the body could use. As a result, it was as if no protein was eaten, and the body had to take its protein from it's own inner sources.

● **LITE** A category for diet food labeling. *See* Label Reading.

m

◆ **MACHINES, EXERCISE** Stationary aerobic exercise devices.

Exercise equipment is a superior way to work out because of the intensity of the workout, but it is important that you gradually build up, so you prevent overexertion. This can be done with *interval training. See* Exercise. Interval Training.

MAGIC BULLET A pill or pill-like formula that is seen as the cure for weight problems. A gimmick. Fad. If you're the kind of dieter who looks for a magic pill for your weight problems, you're not alone. Most of the dieters in the country have experimented with some form of fad, and it takes a lot of failure to cure the habit. Part of it has been created by our culture that promotes fast cures in TV and magazine ads, and it doesn't go away by pretending it doesn't exist. Even scientists are looking for magic pills to end our weight loss problems once and forever. But they know the difference between realistic expectations and false ones. So do you, and yet you still get lured by that magic pill idea. Consider this one — it's a pill-like part of grains — the center or kernel, filled with nutrition and a source of carbohydrates that are significant for weight loss. So there you are, it's the one you've been looking for all along.

MAGIC FORMULA A mix that is seen as the cure for weight loss. Everyone likes to believe in magic, and the entire staff of Walt Disney is there to prove that magic can be a positive part of life. It can be a positive part of weight loss too, if you look for the magic in the right place — your food and exercise.

The best formula for fat burn is the following real food:

Complex Carbs	60%
Lean Protein	20%
Low Fat	20%
Water	2 Quarts
Tab Vitamin/Mineral	1
Exercise	3 x per week/ 30 minutes/session.

This formula would work on Prince Charming, Snow White, Rose Red, Bugs Bunny, Elmur Fudd, Mickey and Minnie Mouse and you.

Who said nature isn't filled with magic?

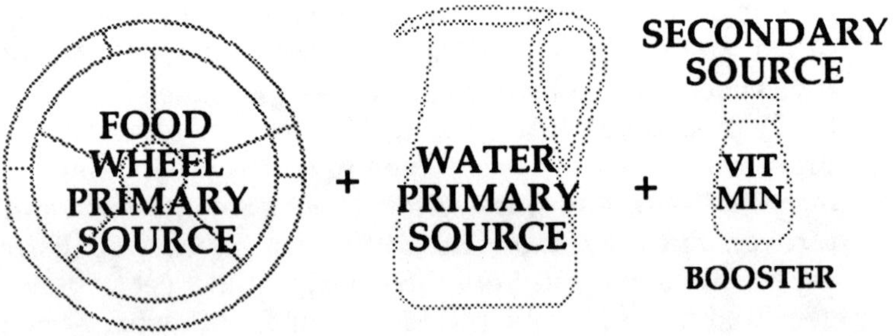

▲ **MAINTENANCE, IDEAL WEIGHT** The energy eaten equals energy burned.

MAINTENANCE CONTINGENCY PLAN:

Set a weight that you will not exceed, in the event that you start letting too much fat creep back into your diet.

SUGGESTED SIGNAL:	8 pounds (Five pounds can be water fluctuations)
PRE-SIGNAL:	5 pounds

If you gain five pounds and it stays there for two or three weeks, review your food wheel and exercise wheel, and use them to evaluate where you're slacking off. Reduce your sodium intake and increase your water drinking, and if the weight stays there, begin to take action. Keep in mind that a 5 pound gain can be muscle, if you are still eating soundly and exercising regularly. The best way to check is the fit of your clothes.

If your weight creeps up to 8 pounds, return to your diet phase for a few weeks. It may be that you need a period of stabilization, if you were carrying extra fat for a long time. Don't see this as a sign of failure! It's just another step to weight maintenance for life. Most people don't understand what maintenance really means. It doesn't mean staying at one precise weight for the rest of your life. It means staying within your weight range for healthy ideal weight.

When you learn to catch your weight before it exceeds eight pounds, your life becomes so much easier. The drama of dieting is diminished, and you are back in shape before it gets out of hand.

Women tend to get more of their fats from cream sauces and sugary foods, so keep an eye on them. Learn to continue your use of non-fattening sauces and gravies after your diet.

IDEAL WEIGHT MAINTENANCE

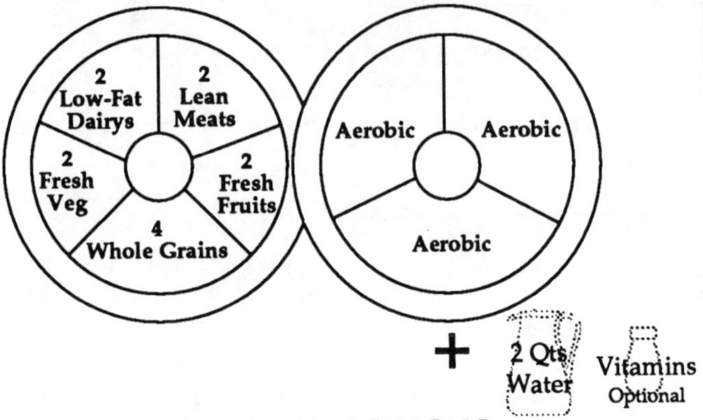

YOUR INPUT IS STRONG
YOUR OUTPUT IS STRONG
THEY WORK TOGETHER TO KEEP YOU LEAN

Your food wheel is ideal. This is the pattern to follow for life. It gives you 50 essential nutrients daily, is high-fiber and low-cholesterol.	Your exercise wheel is ideal. This is the pattern you should use for life. It will keep you burning the food you eat, and it will continue to tone your body. It keeps you lean as you age.

MAINTENANCE AFTER A DIET

YOUR GOAL: Stay balanced! To do that, you increase your calories in the complex carbohydrate group — vegetables, fruits and grains. You can increase your fats, but you should ask yourself why you would want to. Every now and then, you can eat something with more fat or sugar, but why do it on a regular basis. This is what you dreamed of. This is the power to stay lean. Use your ability to increase your fats within the group of high-yielding nutrient foods, not the low-yield processed ones. Keep up your water level. It will keep incoming fat going out. If you have a bowl of ice cream, choose the low fat yogurt kind. Explore the world of food and nutrition that is now available to you. Always meet the minimum on the diet food wheel daily. That will keep you stable.

Men tend to get more of their fat from proteins — those big steak dinners. So keep an eye on your protein that contains hidden fats. A good plan is to stay with the leaner proteins on a regular basis, and only add the fatter ones now and then.

MAINTENANCE MINDSET:

Remember: You weren't born to be fat and to get fat even after you dieted to get lean. You were born to be lean. Babies are born with body compositions in the appropriate balance, and with very little differentiation between male and female babies. Your lifestyle changes your body composition. And your lifestyle can change it back to its ideal state. Sure, it takes a little work, but that's part of the process of learning how to treat yourself right.

If your mind's eye is letting you gain eight extra pounds, and you're letting it happen, take action against the picture of having your fat back. Each time you re-train yourself away from fat, and away from seeing yourself fat, your inner power to stay lean gains more of a foothold. Your brain is a historical organ. It only remembers what you tell it about your needs, desires and wants. If you tell it you are going to regain, and your actions duplicate that feeling, you'll recreate the lifestyle that helped you gain weight. If you want to stop that cycle, you can.

Just start.

If you see yourself gaining eight pounds, start eating according to the diet wheel again and regulate your exercise. The burn off time will be faster.

What difference does it make if it takes two or three burnoff sessions to stabilize yourself. Does that make you feel less successful? It shouldn't. It should make you feel great. That's the strategy that normal-weight people use to keep their weight in line for life. That's successful maintenance.

● **MARGARINE** A food that is more vegetable fat than animal fat (or should be). Butter substitute. *See* Cholesterol.

MEAL REPLACEMENT A formula, usually protein, that is used instead of a regular meal in a diet plan. *See* Supplements. Meal Replacement Diets.

MEAL REPLACEMENT DIETS Plans that use formulas, usually protein, to substitute for meals. The reason protein is the standard formula for meal replacement diets is twofold. Meal replacement diets aim for the lowest calorie ceiling they can get. Fresh fruits, vegetables and grains have minimal fat and calories, so it wouldn't make sense to replace them with a better variety. The protein foods are the ones that contain hidden fat, therefore making a protein with less fat reduces the overall calorie ceiling dramatically. Secondly, protein is mandatory on a diet to preserve your body muscle. A diet would be dangerous for your health without adequate protein. While this makes sense theoretically, in practice these diets don't pay off. It may be that the processed proteins don't have the same metabolic effect and benefits of real protein foods, but this has to be researched. It's also a calorie problem. When you go on very low calorie diets, your metabolism slows down, and you burn less calories overall. Over time, as you continue to eat and burn less calories, your body adjusts to this lower calorie level, and your metabolism is burning at its low point. When you go off the diet, you aren't a good fat burner, and you gain weight fast. If you *must* use a meal replacement plan that is very low in calories, do it under a doctor's care where you can be supervised.

MEDICAL CHECKUP A routine health physical. Whenever you go on a diet, you should precede it with a visit to your doctor, who knows your medical history. You can use the results of your physical to take a look at your food input and energy output to see where you can make improvements. When you go on a diet that is 800 calories or less, it must be doctor-monitored! An 800-

calorie diet (or less) is *serious* restriction, and not usually preferred by doctors as the first, best course. The easiest and best way to diet is with a balanced food plan that meets your daily nutrient needs. That way, you avoid the risks and get double the benefits. And the next time you go for your physical, you'll be healthier as well as slimmer.

▲ **MEDITATION** Mental stillness or calm, achieved through a specific method of relaxation. Also know as transcendental meditation.

Meditation is a process of relaxation that brings your mind and body into a deeply silent state. It's the ideal relaxation, easy to do, and richly rewarding. Advocates say it gives you a new lease on life. It deepens sleep, reduces insomnia and restlessness, and gets you in touch with your inner resources for strength, clarity and self-appreciation.

Meditation Needs:

1. A quiet comfortable place.
2. A fixed time schedule for meditation. The same time every day. The best time is usually the first thing in the morning, since your mind is in a less frenzied state.
3. Uninterrupted time for 10-15 minutes to start.
4. No prescription drugs for 24 hours prior to meditation.
5. No food or beverages 2 hours before meditation.
6. Your own word or mantra sound, that you keep to yourself.
7. The right frame of mind. Don't see meditation as a duty or obligation. You are not being judged or graded on your progress. Trust the process, and don't concern yourself with results. Make it a gift you give yourself each day.

Meditation Goals:

1. Physical Stillness. Find a posture where you can practice remaining still. The one suggested for beginners is sitting in a comfortable chair with your feet flat on the floor, hands resting loosely in your lap. You can also lie on the floor on a rug or mat, but for first-timers it's not recommended, since you can fall asleep. You want a position that will keep you from fidgeting, while allowing you to remain mentally alert.
2. Adjusting to Stillness. Once you begin meditating, urges come over you to shift, scratch and itch, cough or be distracted by outside noises. Part of the process of meditation is to resist all of these urges calmly to achieve mental and physical stillness. Many meditators find that this takes time to learn and pass through. The point is to keep doing it.
3. Experiencing the sound vibrations. Sound is used in meditation for its tranquilizing effect. Since the mind's tendency is to be distracted, the sound also creates focus and the ability to concentrate. The sound that is required is very specific. It must be open and expansive to start, must have resonance and good vibrational power, and it must close at the end to keep the vibrations inside you. The sound OM is the most common mantra, and is considered the perfect sound for meditation. It is a word which combines 3 sounds — AAAA OOOO MMMM, opening with the A sound and closing with the M sound. Many people like to use the word *home* or *calm* for their mantra. The sound or mantra is used with your breathing, and should be used on exhaling, lasting the full length of the exhale.

➡ **How To Meditate**

Assume your position and breathe in and out, using your mantra as you exhale. Repeat the process for 10 minutes to start, and gradually extend the time to 15-20 minutes each session. The more you repeat the meditation, the easier it becomes to go deeper into relaxation.

MEGAVITAMIN Large doses of a particular vitamin or nutrient. Megavitamin therapy is usually used in the case of specific illnesses or conditions which are caused by chronic depletion of vitamins or nutrients. It should never be used as a dietary practice on an unsupervised basis. It can cause serious harm, since excessive intake of one vitamin can imbalance all the others. If you eat a balanced diet, your vitamins and minerals will be provided in your food. If you do not eat a balanced diet, and can't seem to get around to improving your food intake, you can take a balanced vitamin/mineral supplement, but you shouldn't view this as a solution to an inadequate diet.

Your system exists in delicate balance, using your vitamins, minerals and nutrients in harmony. This is particularly true of the amino acids, which recently have been used as vitaminlike supplements on an isolated basis. Tryptophan, for instance was promoted as a sleep aid and taken in handfuls by wired up dieters. The unfortunate result is a rare blood disease, either brought on by, or aggravated by the use of one amino acid in isolation (which may have been contaminated in the factory).

The problem with megavitamin-itis is that it distorts your view of vitamins, minerals and nutrients that occur naturally in foods. If pills are contaminated, or removed from the market, users of the product begin to FEAR the naturally-occurring variety, staying away from food. Hardly a day goes by without some vitamin or mineral being singled out for abuse. This is *not* caused by the use of food as a vitamin/mineral source, but by abuse in pill form, then sadly transferred to food.

Dieters are the population most susceptible to megavitamin hype. Weight is an emotional issue, and the desire is always there for a magic formula or pill to take it all away. It is also part of a problem created by poor diets which promote one enzyme, one vitamin, or one mineral as the cure-all for weight problems. Some of these programs even have doctors names on them, but you should notice, that regardless of the gimmick — the enzyme, vitamin, or mineral usually occurs IN THE PRESENCE OF a calorie-balanced diet. You are being sold a miracle pill idea, when the miracle is really in your food.

This magic cure idea is perpetuated by dieters themselves. The problem is *they sell.* If they didn't sell, companies wouldn't keep producing them. It's up to you, as a dieter, to stop supporting these gimmicks and fads. You owe it to yourself to turn your attention back to real food. That's where the success rates are greater. That's where the only side effects are losing your fat, not inviting other, greater health risks.

The final problem with isolated vitamin or enzyme plans is doubly sad for people with weight problems. They fail, and you continue to gain weight.

METABOLIC RATE Your rate of heat production, measured in specific units, or calories—usually calories per hour, or kilocalories per day (kilocalorie equals 1000 calories). All of your body processes produce heat as a byproduct of chemical reactions which are occurring at all times. Eating, digestion, motion, body maintenance, and metabolism itself release heat. For your heart to beat, a chemical reaction takes place that releases heat. To breathe, a chemical reaction releases heat. This heat can be measured as it escapes your body, and that measurement is your metabolic rate.

There are two ways to measure your metabolic rate, but don't go running to your doctor, because these methods are expensive and reserved for research.

1. There is a machine called a metabolic calorimeter, which measures the amount of heat escaping from

solid bodies. You could be put inside that machine, and your heat production could be measured. This is a very costly and complicated process.

2. Since the first process is costly and complicated, a more practical method was devised. Heat and oxygen have a unique relationship. When heat is released from your body, oxygen is consumed. A liter of oxygen is consumed for every 4.8 kilocalories of heat produced. Therefore, you can measure metabolic rate by measuring the rate of oxygen that is consumed, and calculating the heat from that. It's a back door approach that allowed scientists to calculate thousands of metabolic rates. In this test, if you were a laboratory subject, you would be required to breathe into a mouthpiece or facemask that is hooked up to a device that measures oxygen, Your metabolic rate would be added to the pool of metabolic rates that give dieters all the values for calories, heat expenditure in exercise, and all those measurements in books that are taken so lightly.

Factors that influence your metabolic rate are:

1. Your Age. Your metabolic rate decreases with age, regardless of your sex.
2. Your Sex. Men have a slightly higher metabolic rate than women, because of their higher body muscle content. Women's metabolic rate is slightly lower because of their higher body fat content, needed to insulate a potential baby.
3. Temperature. In colder climates, your metabolic rate is higher. In warmer climates, it's lower. (This may also make antarctica a very popular resort for dieters next year.)
4. Activity Level. The more you move, the higher your metabolic rate.
5. Time of Day. Your metabolic rate slows down toward the end of the day. It goes into a very slow state while

you are sleeping, called a "fasting" state. This means you should not eat your heaviest meals at night, when you can't burn calories as well.

6. Your State of Health or Dis-ease. Your metabolic rate can be affected by certain conditions. Stress will give you a higher metabolic rate, but it will also burn you out faster. Weight will give you a lower metabolic rate. Heavier people have lower metabolic rates per unit of body weight than lighter people. This is caused by the higher body fat content, and lower muscle content, since muscle tissue is the site for fat burning.
7. Food Intake. The food you eat can increase your metabolic rate. This is called Specific Dynamic Action, and you can use that to your advantage. After you eat, your metabolic rate rises for several hours, even if nothing else occurs. The effect is greater after eating low-fat protein and carbohydrates, and last comes fat. This is caused by the biochemical reactions (heat producing) that go on in your cells to process the nutrients derived from food, and to use those nutrients to build up your body.

To discover all these facts about Basal Metabolic Rate, scientists had to find a way to measure it without the variables or interferences , such as individual activity levels, eating styles, and climate. To do this, they measured metabolic rates in resting states and came up with a standard for basal metabolism, or the heat production required for your body to maintain itself on the-most basic level—to keep your lungs functioning, heart beating, eyes opening and closing, ad infinitum.

Basal measurements were taken with the following requirements:

1. The people had to be at rest but not sleeping.
2. The temperature couldn't be too hot or too cold.

3. No food could be eaten 24 hours prior to the test.

In this way, the figures were derived for your body's basic need to maintain itself or keep itself alive, without added activity, temperature differences or internal food processing occurring. This is how the figures for basal metabolic rate were determined. After that, activity levels could be calculated, exercise levels could be tallied, and calorie levels could be determined, by the way they affect basal metabolic rate.

Your daily metabolic rate can be increased by adding on the factors that increase it — more activity, better eating, more exercise. That's how you drive up your metabolic rate to produce more heat and burn more calories daily. That's how you retrain your body not to hold on to its fat.

METABOLISM The biochemistry of life. At all times during the day, thousands of chemical reactions are occurring in your cells. The nutrient molecules from digestion are circulating in your blood, ready to be taken up for metabolic work—repair and maintenance of your entire body system, from your heart to a nerve impulse. Different cells take different nutrients, depending on the jobs they have to do.

For instance, your muscles are made of two different proteins. Cells have to make these muscle proteins, and each one has to be different from each other, and different from the amino acids floating in your bloodstream after digestion. A cell can make some of the amino acids for its new protein by itself, by breaking the bonds of a sugar molecule and converting it to an amino acid. But the cell cannot make eight of the possible amino acids needed for its new protein. It has to get them from you, through your food. The cell takes the amino acid provided from your food, and breaks its bonds, freeing up the amino acids it needs to complete its chain. This metabolic process is called *CATABOLISM*—the breaking down of available compounds.

When the cell makes its new protein and you have some new muscle molecules, this metabolic process is called *ANABOLISM*—the building of new compounds from others. These two processes, anabolism and catabolism are going on simultaneously, all over your body. All of the materials of your body are being created in cells that are breaking down the nutrients from food.

If the amino acid isn't available to the cell, no muscle will be made today. One-half of your body protein is rebuilt every three months by your cells. A blood cell lives for four months, then has to be destroyed and replaced with a new one.

Your body is what you give it on a daily basis.

When the bonds of any molecule are broken, heat is produced. You can't use the heat as energy and it leaves your body. The collective heat from these processes of breaking nutrient bonds to build new materials for your body is your METABOLIC RATE, BASAL. The better you eat, the more you accelerate this process, because the nutrients are there for the cells to take. It takes approximately 60% of your calories to operate these processes, calories you don't store as fat. If you don't provide the nutrients, the reactions don't take place as often or as well, and you burn less calories!

When the bonds of a nutrient are broken, some energy escapes and isn't used by the cell. It's picked up by the chemical ADP (Adenosine Diphosphate) and stored in the bonds of its big sister ATP Adenosine TriPhosphate). This chemical circulates around your body bringing energy where it's needed. Every movement and motion requires that the bonds of ATP be broken, to get the energy out. This releases heat. The heat from these reactions are the heat of your metabolic rate, over the basal rate. If you are active and exercise, you are stimulating many more chemical reactions that release heat. These are calories that don't store.

If you don't do much moving around and don't do much exercise, the excess sugars and amino acids are converted to fat for storage in your adipose tissue. The major sites of adipose tissue are directly beneath your skin, in your abdomen, and in your buttocks. The major storage sites for glycogen (from carbohydrates) is in your liver and in your muscles, to be used for energy, but the carbohydrate stores are small compared to fat.

As time goes by, your adipose mass gets larger from these stores, and your muscle mass has to perform all of the chemical reactions it takes to support that mass and the added pressure on your system. Cells are waiting for nutrients to build their proteins and other body materials but sugars and fatty acids seem to predominate. And there aren't enough vitamins and minerals to get the process activated. The cells sit waiting. No muscle protein is made today, or tomorrow. Your metabolic rate slows down. Your cells don't have the nutrients they need to make new materials. (And that just the protein materials. Your body needs many more).

Dieting and Your Metabolism

When you diet to correct this problem, the first priority is to *provide these nutrients, in the form your body needs*. That may not be the form provided in some of the diets you can find in your neighborhood. But you can find it in the Food Groups. That's the beauty of science. It's based on the energy of metabolism.

MINERALS Organic or inorganic nutrients found in your body and food. Less than 5% of your total body weight is minerals, but their role is crucial. They are part of your body fluids and tissues, protecting your muscle tissue and nervous system. They aid digestion, metabolism, hormone production, help create antibodies, and many are responsible in catalyzing enzymes to facilitate metabolic processes. There are 17 essential minerals, and all of them need to be supplied by your food daily. Some are called *macro-minerals,* because they are present in high amounts in your body (for a mineral) — these are calcium, chlorine, phosphorous, magnesium, sodium and sulfur. They're measured in milligrams (1/1000 gram). Others are called trace minerals, because they are present in your body in very small amounts, but some are very essential. They're measured in micrograms (1/1,000,000 gram).

Best Source for Minerals

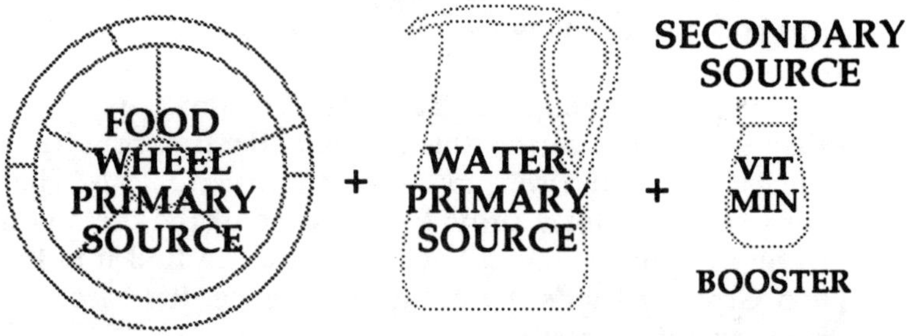

All of your minerals work together, and excesses of one mineral can throw off the balance of the others. Distilled water removes minerals. Excess fiber can bind with minerals, and you excrete them.

When you are on a low-calorie diet, it's essential to take a vitamin/mineral supplement. Otherwise, you get all your minerals from the food group eating plan.

Dictionary of Minerals

ALUMINUM	trace/toxic in excess
BERYLLIUM	Trace/toxic
CADMIUM	trace/toxic
ANTIDOTE — Zinc	
CALCIUM	essential/macro
CHLORINE	essential/macro
CHROMIUM	essential
COBALT	essential
COPPER	essential/trace
FLUORINE	essential/trace
sodium fluoride in water can be harmful	
ANTIDOTE — Calcium	
IODINE	essential/trace
IRON	essential
LEAD	trace/toxic
ANTIDOTE — Zinc	
MAGNESIUM	essential/macro
MERCURY	trace/toxic
MOLYBDENUM	trace/essential
NICKEL	trace/essential
PHOSPHOROUS	essential/macro
POTASSIUM	essential
SELENIUM	trace/essential
SODIUM	essential/macro
SULFUR	essential/macro
VANADIUM	trace/essential
ZINC	trace/essential
OTHERS: BORON, LITHIUM, SILICON, STRONTIUM, TIN, TRITIUM	trace/essential.Their role in nutrition isn't known.

▲ **MIRROR EXERCISES** Techniques for evaluating and changing your negative inner perceptions. Body image issues in a glance. Mirrors are two-dimensional. They do not give you a realistic view of yourself. When you look in the mirror, how you see yourself is a reflection of your inner views about yourself, your weight, and your attitude. How you respond to what you see is a body image issue.

➡ **How To Do A Mirror Image Appraisal**

Stand in front of the mirror in underwear or nude.

What do you look at first?

Your face or your body?

When you look at your body, do you look at your whole body, or parts of your body that are fatter than other parts. Which parts do you look at? The thin parts or fatter parts.

Most people with weight problems tend to look at themselves from the neck up first, and not at their whole image in the mirror.

Most people with weight problems also tend to look at *parts* rather than the whole image. They will single out their heavier parts and forget to look at their slimmer parts. Or they will avoid their heavier parts and concentrate on their thin parts. Either way, this is fragmented thinking, because it singles out specific problems, whether you look at the problems or avoid them. To have this fragmented image, you don't necessarily have to be overweight. Many thin people look at themselves as parts that need to be fixed, rather than as a person in the mirror who is unique in life.

CREATING A POSITIVE MIRROR IMAGE

Your view in the mirror is subjective and often fragmented. To make your weight goals more objective, get a notebook and pen. Stand in front of the mirror again.

First, look at your whole self, taking in your height, length of your trunk and legs, and even your feet. Turn a shoulder to the mirror, so you can get a more three-dimensional effect.

Next, objectively evaluate what areas you would like to change with weight loss. List them in your notebook. Hips, buttocks, belly. Make the list as short or as long as you need.

Now look in the mirror again and study each of the parts you listed. If you listed your hips, look at your hips. Write down the first thought that comes to your mind about your hips, using these guidelines:

My hips look like ________________________.
This makes me feel________________________.

Use this format for each of the body parts you listed Be honest. This record is for you. You may continue to write the things you start feeling, and you can write as much as you like. But try to answer the two questions for each body part you listed.

After you are finished, stand in front of the mirror again.

Read your response to the mirror for each part.

Then change each negative response to a positive one.

For instance:

My hips look like tankers.

CHANGE: My hips look like the hips of a strong woman (man).

My hips allow me to turn quickly. They support my

upper body. I used to hold my baby on my right hip when I was shopping. Say anything you want to switch your response to a positive response.

Follow this procedure with all the parts you listed.

How does it make you feel to say something nice about yourself?

If it makes you uncomfortable, ignore the discomfort. Practice this exercise again tomorrow and try to feel good and light when you say something nice about a body part you think you don't like.

If it makes you feel light and surprised with the feeling, you've accomplished this exercise. But that doesn't mean negative thoughts won't creep back in. Every time you think something negative about a body part, use the positive substitution process, until the negative feeling lets go.

If you don't believe what you're saying, it doesn't make any difference. Your brain is a recorder of your responses and feelings. It will repeat back to you what you feel and see. It may take time to get your brain used to the idea that you are not insulting yourself regularly. But it will learn it. And you will lift a great weight off your self image. This will give you support to achieve your goals.

WHOLE SELF APPRECIATION

Stand in front of the mirror in underwear or nude and look at yourself.

Absolutely and unequivocally love who you see. Say *I love you* to the person in the mirror. Tap the mirror to assert it. Repeat it until you believe it. If you don't believe it the first time you do it, keep doing it. Eventually, you will feel what it feels like to love yourself in the mirror. It does not matter how much fat you have, or where you have it, how long you've had it, who likes it or doesn't, or if you ever intend to let go of it. This has nothing to do with external weight. This has to do with you as a person in the world. You are uniquely and distinctly you, and that is uniquely and distinctly beautiful. Do this exercise at least 2 times a day, once in the morning and before bed at night.

Every time your mind wanders to a part, stop it.

Breath deeply and look at your whole self again and love you.

You may get a number of negative-sounding thoughts to try to take you away from your purpose, which is learning to love yourself exactly like you are. You can explore those thoughts at your leisure, because they will reveal interesting reasons why you think you don't like yourself. Always assume power over the thought. For instance, you might look in the mirror and say I love you to yourself, and in the back of your mind you'll hear: *No you don't.* Or,*You shouldn't wear your hair that way.* Or, *You're getting crows feet.* Or even, *You never do what I tell you to do.* Or even, You don't deserve something.

You can listen to these thoughts, but realize that they don't own you anymore. They are trained thoughts. They came from someone or came somehow in the process of life. You do not have to go through years of psychoanalysis to stop those thoughts. You can change them every time they come up. You can change them in the mirror every time you look at yourself. When you do this, it begins to change you. Gradually, you stop dealing from negative places and negative viewpoints, and you begin to look at things differently. You begin to look at things almost as if you were a child amused with life again. This is the person you really want to own, that amused child grown up. That child was born to love herself/himself. When you deal with yourself from a place that is loving and positive, you can accomplish anything you set your mind to.

MODERATION The midpoint between extremes. A behavior key for extreme thinkers. Dieters tend to think in extremes, especially ones who have been trained to do it by deprivation diets. A diet is seen as a short-term affair that is unpleasant, therefore, the sooner it's over the better. Unfortunately, this kind of thinking leads to failure and weight regain. The reasoning is: if a diet can take off 10 pounds in a month, then stricter dieting will take off 20.

FOOD. Extreme thinkers see foods in two categories. Good Foods/Bad Foods, Their Foods/My Foods. Diet foods are good, all other foods are bad. The only trouble is, each diet has foods they say are good, and others say are bad. This leads to food confusion, and generates anxiety about food. Every time a new food arrives in the supermarket, it's seen as a curse or a cure. This also leads to abnormal eating habits, which remove whole categories of food from the daily plan. Often carbohydrates are removed from diets, when the natural complex carbohydrates are the best fat burners and fiber sources for dieting.

Moderation means developing a whole new philosophy about food. Food is your energy, and primary source of nutrients, and it's not the food that gives you trouble, it's how you use it. Using food wisely gives you more variety and flexibility in your diet, it opens up a world of pleasures, instead of a limited menu of food monotony. A new relationship with food is like a new lease on life.

PROGRAMS. Extreme thinkers tend to choose extreme programs, the stricter the better. The more miserable you are on a diet, the more it re-inforces the idea that you should be punished for having weight. That leads you to want sweet treats and fats for reward. This also separates the "diet" from real life, as if they have nothing to do with each other. You bring this separation into your daily routine and habits, and before you know it, your perspective on other things begins to change too.

Moderation lifts you out of this pattern. You begin to see extremes for what they are-stress promoting habits. Your daily life should be less stressed on your diet, and there should not be such a gap between the diet phase and maintenance. When you practice moderate habits during your diet, you wind up at ideal weight with the skills you need to stay there. That leads to a healthier outlook on everything in life.

EXERCISE. Extreme thinkers go all out on exercise or don't do it at all. Everything on the weekend and nothing during the week. Jump in fast and get out fast. This can cause injury, and it can use the wrong kind of energy for your exercise. You can be doing most of your activity on an anaerobic level—not getting oxygen uptake.

Moderation means that you gradually increase your activity and aerobic exercise, learning to experiment with options, to find choices that give you pleasure, not strain, pulled muscles and fatigue. This is the original intent of exercise, physical and cardiovascular conditioning, and it makes everything run more smoothly in your life.

MONOUNSATURATED A type of unsaturated fat, or OK fat. *See* Cholesterol.

MUSCLE Body protein or muscle tissue. Also called lean body mass. *See* Weight.

n

▲ **NEGATIVE THINKING** A mindset that subverts your success. The solution to this is found in positive-self statements. Every time you express a negative, or think in the negative, you change it to its positive counterpart. You don't even have to believe it. It works anyway. For examples, *See* Mirror Exercises.

▲ **NETWORKING** A support skill for dieting and weight maintenance. Networking means finding booster systems to help you through the rough spots while you are dieting and trying to stay fit. Going it alone can be difficult, but is not impossible. Networks of friends, organizations, or even positive thinking tapes can help you get the incentive you need to keep going. *See* Buddy System.

◆ **NORDIC TRACK** Stationary aerobic machine. Simulated Cross-Country Skiing.

Benefits:

- Best cardiovascular training.
- Best calorie-burning exercise.
- No orthopedic injury; no shock to joints and muscles.
- Works upper and lower body (especially buttocks); can adjust tension for greater strength building and

higher intensity.
- Builds coordination and rhythm.

Guidelines:
- Slip feet into stirrups on skiis, which glide along track.
- Lean slightly forward, balancing pelvis against pelvic cushion.
- Grasp handles on arm pulley.
- Position arms and legs in opposite positions (i.e., left leg forward, right leg back — toe bends up — right arm pulled up, left arm pulled back).
- Then switch positions, gliding opposite leg forward and simultaneously pulling arm pulley, switching arm positions.
- If you struggle with either leg or arm movement, decrease tension on either or both gauges.
- The goal is to develop a comfortable, gliding stride. The opposition of arm and leg movement keeps your balance while you lean forward against the pelvic cushion.
- Handle bars are also attached so you can start out just learning leg coordination, yet in the long run, it's easier to balance when the machine is used as designed with arms and legs in opposition. It's a natural stride, like walking. Don't outthink your stride, just glide! *See* Exercise.

NORMAL WEIGHT Your ideal weight, based on height/weight tables. This gives you a weight *range,* not simply one set weight, or one number for ideal pounds. Some people are comfortable with a higher weight, and as long as it doesn't involve weight-related risks, a higher weight in your weight range would still be safe and normal. *See* Ideal Weight Body.

● **NUTRIENT DENSITY** The ratio of nutrition-to-food-unit, the energy food provides. Eating for nutrient density means getting the most nutrient power for the least calories. For instance:

1/2 CUP FRESH STRAWBERRIES 30 calories in addition to standard nutrients	1/2 CUP FROZEN STRAWBERRIES (SYRUP) 125 calories standard nutrients plus empty calories (sugar)
NUTRIENT DENSITY	CALORIE DENSITY
1 BAKED POTATO MEDIUM 125 calories standard nutrients and trace fat	6 FRENCH FRIES 125 calories standard nutrients, excess fat perhaps saturated fat
NUTRIENT DENSITY	CALORIE DENSITY

Choosing your foods for nutrient density is the easiest way to stay satisfied on a diet while you lose fat.

● **NUTRIENT NEEDS** The carbohydrates, protein, fat, vitamins, minerals and water required to maintain your body and burn fat better. RDAs—required daily allowances. The best source for complete nutrient satisfaction on a daily basis is the Food Groups, which gives you 50 essential nutrients, along with your daily vitamins and minerals in an easy-to-use system. It includes complex carbohydrates for energy and fiber, low-fat proteins for energy, muscle protection and balanced amino acids, and calcium for strong bones. Anything less is not the best. *See* Food Group.

● **NUTRIENTS** Nourishment that produces energy or aids in the production of energy. The essential nutrients for your body energy and calorie burn are:

CARBOHYDRATES PROTEIN FAT VITAMINS MINERALS WATER	Body nutrients are derived from food nutrients. Food nutrients become nutrient supplements, such as vitamins and minerals It all starts with food. That's the source to return to.

EASIEST AND BEST SOURCE FOR DAILY NUTRIENT INSURANCE AND FAT BURN.

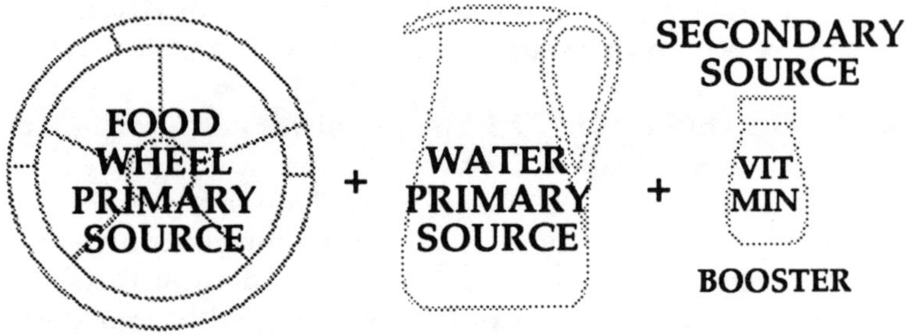

THIS IS IDEAL NUTRITION AND IDEAL NUTRITION-FOR-FAT-BURN. THERE'S NO BETTER WAY TO DIET. *See* Food Groups.

● **NUTRITION** Achieving daily nutrient status at optimum. That means meeting your recommended daily allowances for protein, carbohydrates, fats, vitamins, minerals and water. *See* Nutrients. Food Groups.

O

OBESITY Excess weight to the degree of 20-30% over ideal body weight. Obesity is generally regarded as a disease, since excess body weight over 30% of ideal weight usually involves other complications such as diabetes and hypertension. However, people can be obese, without any overt signs or symptoms of disease.

Obesity is a disease of malnutrition, not necessarily overeating. Studies have shown that obese people can eat the same amount of calories as a normal-weight person, but still gain weight. Part of this problem is due to the oversized fat mass that steals nutrients and keeps the body malnourished or imbalanced nutritionally. Part of the problem is activity — which is decreased with obesity. The heavier you get, the more you tend to slow down and avoid exercise. As a result, you burn less calories. And one of the biggest factors is the content of your daily diet — it is often imbalanced, and thrown off in the direction of sugar and fat.

On the next page, you'll see the problems in context, and how to resolve them. While obesity is a higher degree of weight gain than *overweight*, the problems with food and activity are similar, and the solution is the best one for any weight problem.

OVERWEIGHT & OBESITY

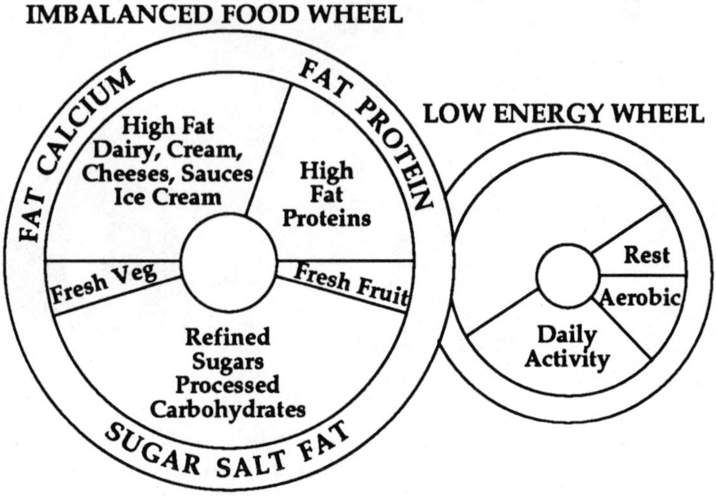

Your INPUT is not in balance
Your ACTIVITY doesn't increase your OUTPUT
The two combine to make your INPUT exceed your OUTPUT
You store more calories than your burn

Your food wheel is not balanced. Even if you get your baseline nutrition, it is depleted or overshadowed by poorer energy sources, like sugar, fat and sodium. Stress depletes your nutrients even more. Your fiber intake is low and fat doesn't mobilize. Your metabolism is slow, so you gain weight even if you eat less. It's a cycle that continues to escalate until you balance your food wheel.

Your activity level is not sufficient to burn the calories you eat. Because you carry fat, you tire easily and exercise seems like a chore, so you put it off. The more you sit, the more you eat, the more you eat, the more you gain. Even when you limit your calories, you still gain, because your body composition is tilted in the direction of fat. If you lost muscle on a poor diet, this compounds your problem, because it helps you to store fat instead of burn it.

YOUR GOAL: Fix your food wheel first, because that will give you more nutrient energy for more activity. Begin with a low-impact aerobic program and work your way up to greater exercise levels as you lose your excess fat.

IDEAL DIET WEEK

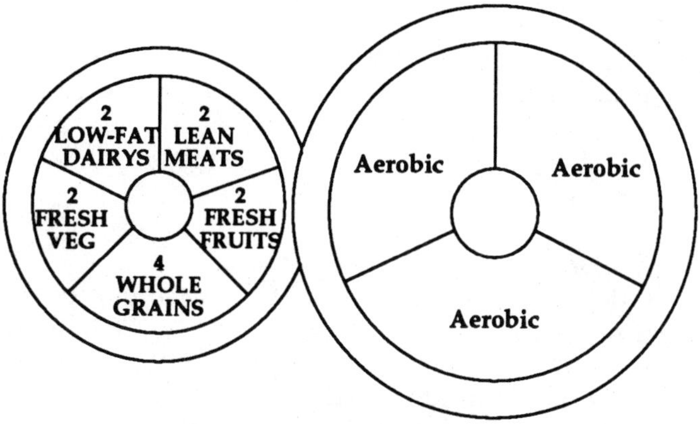

Your INPUT Drives up your OUTPUT
Your ACTIVITY Drives up your OUTPUT
RESULT: Your OUTPUT exceeds your INPUT
You burn more than you eat

Your food burns calories too from thermogenesis — the heat of eating. The wheel provides the 50 essential nutrients you need to feed your metabolism, to activate its chemical action to repair, rebuild and maintain all of your body processes, from the largest organ to the smallest cell. When you take the wheel to its low-fat format, the result is: fat burns and burns.

Your 30 minute aerobic routine, 3 x per week drives up your metabolism to burn more calories (15%+). It also builds muscle, the vital body protein you lose from poor dieting and need to rebuild, in order to be a better fat burner for life. These factors combine to revive your sluggish metabolism, align your body composition, and set you up with the status you need to stay lean after your diet.

Overall result: While fat is burning, muscle is restored. You get superior weight loss and a body composition to match. In maintenance, you will be able to raise your calorie level without regaining.

YOUR GOAL: TO GET BACK IN BALANCE

● **OILS** Vegetable oils, or unsaturated fats. These are considered good sources of fat because they help remove cholesterol, rather than add to it. *See* Cholesterol.

OSTEOPOROSIS Reduction in bone mass and density, brittle bones. The more weight you have, the greater your tendency for osteoporosis, from the pressure of weight, dietary deficiencies and sedentary tendencies that go along with weight.

The major causes of osteoporosis are:

1. Calcium-deficient diet, usually over a long period of time. When you eat too little calcium, your body takes the calcium it needs from your bones. These losses can't be restored to your bones, except by meeting your daily calcium needs in your food.
2. Lack of weight-bearing exercise. Calcium absorption is increased with exercise, and lack of it means less calcium absorption. Weight-bearing exercises are ones where your body bears the weight, such as walking (instead of swimming). This increases your bone strength along with your calcium absorption.
3. Calcium-phosphorus imbalance. You need equal amounts of calcium and phosphorous for calcium to absorb properly. How do you get it without worrying? Balanced meals from the food groups.
4. Intestinal absorption problems. This may be the result of dietary deficiencies of phosphorous, Vitamin D, and Protein along with lack of exercise, or it can be caused by underlying medical conditions and hormonal issues.
5. Cigarette smoking inhibits calcium absorption, along with many other nutrients. A good reason to stop. (If you don't intend to stop, you need more calcium, exercise and vitamins/minerals than a non-smoker.)

The primary nutrients needed for calcium absorption are: Vitamins B12, C, D, E, Copper, Fluoride, Magnesium,

Phosphorous and Protein. *See* Calcium.
CAUTION! Dieters are notorious for casually eliminating milk and other dairy products from their diets, thinking that they're major sources of fat. Don't diet if you're going to do that! Use 1% or 2% lowfat milk and other lowfat dairy products and eat plenty of vegetables daily to get your calcium requirements. What's a good body without good bones.

OUTPUT Calories burned, specifically on a daily basis. Output is one half of the energy scale that determines your weight, or weight regulation. The balanced state is:

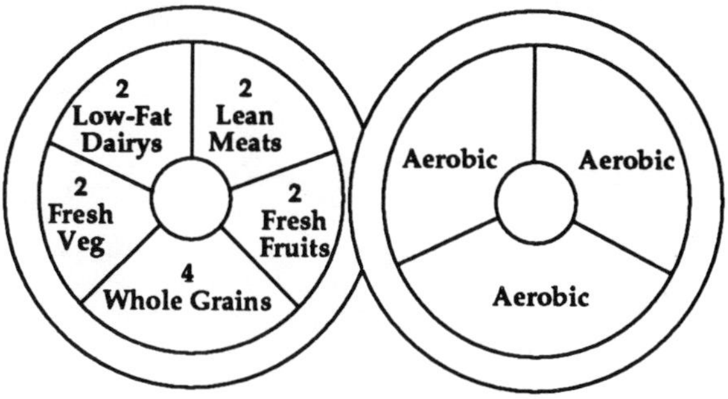

Input Equals Output
Calories Eaten Equal Calories Burned

Output is a combination of heat producing processes that include running your body shop to keep you living, activities you do in your everyday life, and exercise you add on for greater heat production and calorie burn. *See* Exercise and Metabolic Rate for the total picture.

OXYGEN UPTAKE The ability of your blood to pick up and carry oxygen. Since oxygen is vital to all body processes and increases fat burn, increasing your oxygen uptake is important. This can be accomplished with exercise and deep breathing exercises. Relaxation and

Meditation can also improve oxygen uptake, since they relax your body and that naturally causes you to breath more deeply. *See* Exercise. Breathing. Relaxation. Meditation.

P

● **PECTIN** A soluble fiber. It prevents blood sugar swings and lowers blood cholesterol. *See* Fiber.

▲ **PERFECTIONIST THINKING** Needing everything to be ideal, or your perception of ideal. This is a trap. It's like driving to your vacation with the map in your lap, and shades down on the windows of your car. You think you're in control, but if you had to stop and spend the afternoon in a strange town, you'd completely lose your grounding. Needing perfection can prevent you from trying something, because you think you already know how it goes. And it can prevent you from succeeding, because life has a way of putting obstacles in your path. Flexibility is the only way to bypass obstacles and get on with your priorities with both feet on the ground. Dieters who set goals that have to be met by a certain date, regardless of the stress, are often perfectionist thinkers. You want to do it once, perfectly, and never again. The trouble is, it backfires. You do it once and perfectly, and you have to do it again because you regain. You don't have the habits you need to deal with all the changing situations of daily life. All you learned were the habits to lose weight in isolation.

The best route to ideal weight is to set standards that are realistic to live with, instead of ones that make your daily life so rigid that a minor crisis can throw off your diet. It takes the pressure off you and makes the process more interesting. Then, if you're caught in a strange town on the way to your vacation, you know how to eat in a restaurant there as well as anywhere, and you know how to find the high school track there as well as anywhere. You've learned how to be flexible. To adapt.

◆ **PHYSICAL ACTIVITY** A means to burn calories. *See* Exercise.

▲ **PLATEAU** A weight you reach during dieting that you can't seem to get below. Often this weight is the last 10 pounds, but a plateau can occur at any time in the weight loss phase.

It's a sign to review your food and exercise patterns.

➡ **How To Overcome A Plateau**

There are two basic steps to overcoming a plateau:

1. Review your food. Keep a food diary for a week to see if fat and sugar are creeping into your diet, while fiber is falling out. Check your carbohydrate, fat and protein levels to see if they are up to par for the best fat burning. Make sure you're not skipping WATER. Make sure you're taking your vitamin/mineral supplement. If you find out that your food intake is perfect, you *can* make an effort to reduce the fat content to a lower level. This will increase the fat that is taken from storage. But don't reduce any other servings in your diet. Less is not best when it comes to nutrition and fat burn. Less means less weight loss, from a reduced metabolism.
2. Review your exercise. If you are loyally exercising three times per week for 30 minutes per session, then you will have to add a low-impact aerobic exercise to your program too. You can take a one hour walk each night to drive up your calorie output.

The combination of these two factors will take you

over the plateau.

Plateaus On Low Calorie Diets

If you are on a very low calorie diet, you've got a problem, and it won't be easy to resolve, but you can do it. You have to go OFF the very low calorie diet and on to a full food program of at least 1200 calories, and you have to put up with the water weight that you will occur in the first week or so. If you stay on the low calorie diet, you may stop losing weight all together. The only way to drive up your metabolism is to reintroduce food, while continuing to exercise and trust in the fat burning effects of real food. This also means that you can't go back to rapid weight loss diets for quick results. You've gotten your metabolism down to such a low ebb that another rapid weight loss diet may cause you to regain beyond your expectations. Don't cheat your body of it's natural potential to use food for fat burn. Follow a balanced diet formula and keep your fat intake as low as you can. Fat loss will happen. Be prepared to wait for it. Celebrate the fact that you've finally broken the habit of rapid weight loss while you're waiting. It's the plateau for a new life.

POLYUNSATURATED A type of unsaturated fat, or OK fat. *See* Cholesterol.

▲ **POSITIVE SELF TALK** A self-strengthening technique. The simple key is to change every negative thing you say to yourself and about yourself to its positive counterpart. *See* Mirror Exercises and Rationalizations for examples.

▲ **POSITIVE THINKING** A success-oriented outlook. This means more than a good attitude going into a diet. It means developing skills that enhance your overall perspective on life. A diet is a part of life, not a separate time away from life. The more lifelike that your diet is, the better you will be able to adapt to ideal weight maintenance, which means eating well for life. The skill of positive-self-talk is a vital one, along with Imagery and Relaxation. For examples of how to do it. *See* Relaxation. Imagery. Mirror Exercises. Rationalizations.

● **POTASSIUM** An essential mineral. Potassium is 5% of the total mineral content of your body, and its role is crucial. In partnership with sodium, potassium regulates the fluid balance on both sides of your cell walls.

Sodium & Chloride

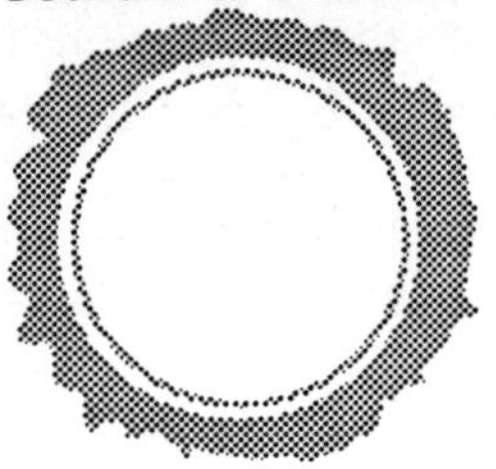

EXTRACELLULAR FLUID

Potassium & Phosphate

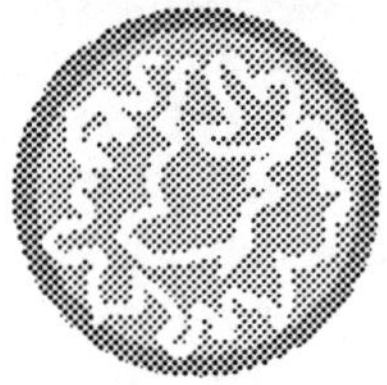

INTRACELLULAR FLUID

Water is the medium for all of your body's reactions. Your cells are surrounded by water and contain water. They're the sites for metabolism and building body compounds. Keeping the sodium/potassium balance is vital to a healthy life.

The recommended daily doses of sodium and potassium are:

SODIUM	POTASSIUM
1,100-3,300 mg/daily	1,800-5,600 mg, daily

Sodium excess is one of the major problems in diets. These excesses cause potassium losses through urine. Excessive use of sugar, alcohol and caffeine can also add to potassium losses. This upsets the balance of sodium and potassium and inhibits the benefits of potassium.

These benefits include:

- healthy nerve impulses and muscle contractions
- conversion of glucose to glycogen for storage
- efficient metabolism
- efficient enzyme reactions
- synthesis of muscle protein from amino acids
- normalized heartbeat
- healthy oxygen supply to brain
- healthy skin
- acid/alkaline balance
- stimulation of kidneys to secrete toxins

SODIUM/POTASSIUM BALANCE

SODIUM — Daily Dose 1,100-3,300 mg

POTASSIUM — 1,800-5,600 mg

AVOID

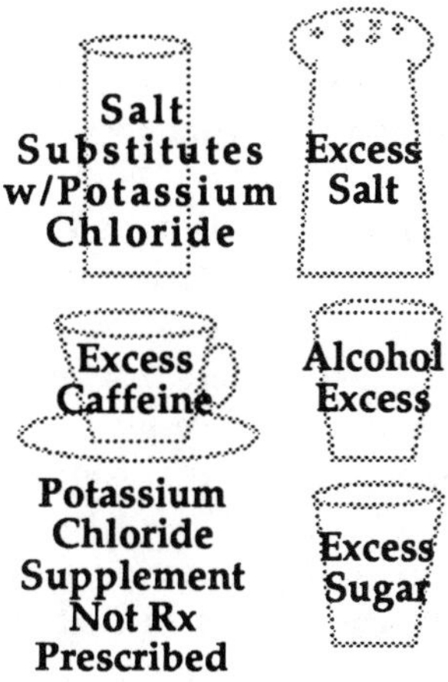

HIGH POTASSIUM FOODS

1 Potato (especially skin)	556 mg
1 cup	
Grapefruit Juice	420
Orange Juice	503
Tomato Juice	549
Prune Juice	602
Skim Milk	355
1 Half Cup	
Banana	221
Broccoli	207
Brussel Sprouts	212
Lentils	249
Squash	473
2 Ounces	
Tuna in water	158
Chicken (skinless)	246
Lean Beef	292

Potassium is usually lost through perspiration or excessive sweating. Refined sugars make your urine alkaline and this means mineral instability. Other causes of potassium deficiency are:

- existing on starvation diets
- use of diuretics
- excessive vomiting
- malnutrition
- diarrhea
- injuries, burns or surgery

Potassium supplements are not recommended as a solution, except in serious cases. The best source is daily replacement of potassium in your food. Potassium supplements contain potassium chloride which can cause bowel lesions, and corrode your intestinal lining. The FDA set the following regulations on potassium chloride:

- tablets with more than 100 mg of potassium chloride must be given under a doctor's supervision
- liquids with more than 20 mg of potassium chloride must be given under a doctor's supervision.

There are rare cases where misuse of potassium supplements along with liquid protein diets, led to death. While this isn't the average situation, it's vital to keep in mind, especially for dieters.

Potassium chloride can be found in salt substitutes, which is why they should not be used without your doctor's approval. Often potassium chloride is used as a flavoring agent, flavor enhancer, stabilizer, thickening agent, or for acid control. Read the labels in order to limit your intake of potassium chloride. Turn to real food, the richest source of potassium, and the natural way to keep your sodium/potassium ratio in line. If you are on a very low calorie diet that is high in sodium, this can deplete your potassium and create weakness, headaches, poor reflexes, saggy muscles, nervousness, and irregular heartbeats.

POUNDS Weight. *See* Weight.

POWDERED PROTEIN A protein supplement used as a meal replacement in a diet plan. *See* Supplements. Meal Replacements.

POWDERED PROTEIN DIETS Programs that use protein supplements in powder form as meal replacements. *See* Supplements. Meal Replacements.

PRESERVATIVES Chemicals used to prevent spoilage in processed foods. *See* Additives.

● **PROCESSED FOODS** Factory versions of real food. Also called refined foods. The most common features of processed foods are high sugar, high salt, high fat, low fiber, high additives, little texture and low nutrition. Even when they're fortified, these foods can't match the fat-burning effects of fresh food. The typical combination of ingredients in processed foods is the formula for storing fat. *See* Sugar.

● **PROTEIN** The word protein comes from a Greek word that means "of first importance." It is a constituent of every cell, and the functional element in glandular secretions, enzymes, and hormones. Protein is essential for tissue growth and repair, regulation of your fluid balance, and stimulation of antibody formation to combat infections.

It is particularly critical for dieters who are cutting back on calories to consider the quality and quantity of protein they need to meet daily requirements.

Proteins are complex substances made up of a series of amino acids or structural building blocks that are chemically bound together. There are 20 or more different amino acids that occur naturally, with the amino acid combinations creating the nature of different proteins. This is the same as forming different words from different combinations of letters. If you were in the middle of the ocean in a sinking boat with a plane flying overhead, and you had only six flag letters to signal the plane, you might spell R-E-S-C-U-E or S-E-C-U-R-E. The arrangement of the letters is of first importance. It's the same with amino acid combinations that form proteins.

Some combinations of amino acids are essential, some are not. Essential amino acids are the ones that cannot be made by your body and therefore must be obtained from your food. The foods that contain all of the essential amino acids in the proper proportions are good-quality proteins, or complete proteins. Animal sources of protein—meat, fish, fowl, eggs, and dairy products—are complete, with the exception of gelatin. Plant proteins, such as grains, beans, fruits, and vegetables, are incomplete, because they lack one or more of the essential amino acids or have insufficient amounts.

You can combine the "incomplete" plant proteins, such as beans, dried peas, lentils, nuts, and seeds, with complementary proteins, such as grains, potatoes, and corn, to form a complete source of protein. This is mandatory for vegetarians to insure adequate protein intake. Many people think there is no such thing as a fat vegetarian, but in fact, vegetarians often eat too much fat, since vegetable protein sources include seeds and nuts, which are high-fat foods. Eating too much food fat adds up to body fat, no matter whose calculator you use. If you are a non-red-meat vegetarian, you might consider eating only low-fat fish and fowl, instead of cheese for protein, to avoid excess fat. If you are a no-meat vegetarian, you might rely on soy, bean and grain casseroles and soups. It is essential for you to get your protein daily and cut out the high-fat cheeses and nuts.

Red-meat-eaters must also be cautious of fat. The most common sources of protein are meats and cheeses, but the best sources for fat loss are the lowest-fat meats and cheeses. In fact, meat is the major source of fat in the average American diet. If you are a red meat eater, you would be wise to switch to the lower-fat fowl and fish and use red meat as a protein source less frequently.

Protein Truths & Falsehoods

It is a common misconception that you can eat a lot of protein without gaining weight. This way of thinking stems largely from the high-protein diets, which were supposedly good fat burners. When high-protein diets first came out, they were well received because people dropped weight fast. Actually, they were loosing weight simply because they were eating fewer overall calories, but eating a lot of protein felt like more eating, mostly because of the fat and bulky quality of meat. Even after the death scares from high-protein liquid diets, many people forgot that the false notions about protein came out of a decade that supported fast weight loss with high protein.

It's time to erase all the faulty information and start fresh. Not only does excess protein store as fat, but when you fill your diet primarily with protein, you are stripping away something else, and usually that's carbohydrates, your main brain food. When you eat a high-protein diet without protecting your daily dairy need, you are inviting calcium leeching from your bones and could wind up with bone deformities or osteoporosis. To stay safe, remember, anything eaten to excess is a dangerous practice.

On the flip side of the coin, protein deficiencies are the last thing a dieter wants. When you do not have enough protein in your diet, your body will break down your muscle tissue in order to meet its protein needs and perform its basic functions. These muscle losses can be life threatening if prolonged. Muscle is what you should gain on your diet.

Another false belief about protein exists among

athletes. Strenuous exercise does not require — and is not enhanced by — increased intake of protein. Rather, you need an increase in the total amount of calories you eat in the form of carbohydrates to meet the energy demands of higher levels of output through exercise.

Your ideal body weight is measured by the amount of lean body mass or muscle you have, and it can never be ideal unless you have enough muscle. During weight loss, you need adequate protein in order to protect your muscle, and insure that you lose only fat.

PSMF Protein Sparing Modified Fast. A diet designed for morbid obesity. The term *sparing* doesn't mean that it uses food protein sparingly, rather that it relies on protein as a primary energy source, since protein is necessary to *spare* or save your body's lean muscle tissue, which is too often lost on a diet. The PSMF is a low calorie diet that was developed specifically for use in medical settings for people who were very severely obese, facing medical risks that endangered their lives. For this reason, the rapid weight loss was justified, because the weight itself was life threatening. However, commercial imitations of this *type* of diet began to appear in the consumer marketplace, and have been used for minor weight loss and mild obesity. In these cases, the diet is not used safely and isn't justified. The PSMF should only be administered under a doctor's supervision, and it is generally agreed that the diet should be restricted to extreme cases of obesity.

▲ **PSYCHOLOGICAL HUNGER** *Desire* for food, as opposed to a *need* for food. *See* Hunger.

q

▲ QUICK FIX MENTALITY

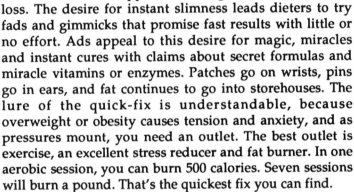

Wanting instant solutions, immediate results. A band-aid approach to weight loss. The desire for instant slimness leads dieters to try fads and gimmicks that promise fast results with little or no effort. Ads appeal to this desire for magic, miracles and instant cures with claims about secret formulas and miracle vitamins or enzymes. Patches go on wrists, pins go in ears, and fat continues to go into storehouses. The lure of the quick-fix is understandable, because overweight or obesity causes tension and anxiety, and as pressures mount, you need an outlet. The best outlet is exercise, an excellent stress reducer and fat burner. In one aerobic session, you can burn 500 calories. Seven sessions will burn a pound. That's the quickest fix you can find.

One of the difficulties about a quick-fix mentality is how you limit your options and deplete your health. When you want to lose weight *fast*, you choose diets that promise 7-10 pounds of weight loss per week. They are the same diets that caused weight regain that is rounder all over. But because you believe that *fast* weight loss is acceptable, you never get to the safer programs, because the safe programs don't make false claims, so they don't sound exciting to you.

Do yourself a favor The next time the urge comes over you to order a gimmick or program that promises fast results, remind yourself that they *mean both fast weight loss,* and *fast weight regain.* Then go for a walk, or do 15-minutes of a relaxation exercise. Afterwards, congratulate yourself for breaking an unhealthy habit! *See* Food Groups, for guidelines to create a healthy habit of eating for life.

r

◆ **RACQUETBALL** Skill sport aerobic exercise. *See* Exercise.

RAPID WEIGHT LOSS Weight loss that exceeds 2-3% of your body weight per week. If you go on a diet and lose 5-7 pounds in a week, that's rapid weight loss. Most of your losses are water in the first week, but after a few weeks, more of your losses will be muscle. On the average rapid weight loss diet, you don't lose a significant amount of fat, compared to your total weight loss. Most rapid weight loss diets show wide fluctuations in weight loss, if you stay on them for a long time. The first few weeks you lose 5-7 pounds and it may keep up for a few more weeks, then suddenly the weight loss drops to a lower level. That's because your body has adjusted to living on fewer calories, and it will try to hoard the limited energy it's getting. The most common problems with rapid weight loss are muscle losses that cause you to regain weight, bouts of binge eating after the diet, and hunger that doesn't seem to turn off. The weight you regain is rounder or plumper-looking than you were before using the rapid weight loss plan, because you are regaining fat fast, and you have less muscle, which is needed for tone.

Habit patterns are a special concern after rapid weight loss diets. In order to develop a diet that takes weight off fast, the food plan must be very restricted, and this leads to good food/bad food attitudes in dieters. A re-entry phase is necessary after a very restricted diet, to teach you how to cope with more food options, but it's often too late, since the habits learned during dieting were not supportive of food variety and learning how to choose foods wisely. The most common habit that emerges after severe food restriction is to EAT and EAT, similar to the behavior after famine.

The faster you lose your weight, the harder it will be to maintain your weight loss. If you are very obese and in your doctor's care, the difficulties with rapid weight loss can be managed and monitored, but that doesn't mean that they won't be there. If you are not in your doctor's care, you shouldn't be on a rapid weight loss diet. *See* Yo Yo Syndrome.

RATIONALIZATIONS Reasons or excuses to postpone self-care, such as weight loss and stress management. Rationalizations and excuses usually take the form of "I don't..." or "I can't...". A simple change of perspective from negative to positive can turn your rationalizations into positive action. To do this, you use *affirmations*, or positive self-statements.This process removes your own defenses, and helps you learn how to solve problems creatively

PROBLEM: I need to lose weight. Therefore I need to diet and exercise.

RATIONALIZATIONS	AFFIRMATIONS
I don't have time	I don't need extra time. I just have to use my time differently. 15 minutes a day for food review, 15 minutes a day for self-strengthening, 30 minutes every other day for exercise. Where will I get the time? I'll take it from negative

	time. The time I take to think I can't is easily 30 minutes a day. So I'll start now.
I don't have the energy.	Getting better daily nutrition will give me more energy. Exercise will give me more energy. So I'll just start, in order to get more energy.
I don't have support.	Eating better and exercising will be very supportive. In addition, I can add further support with imagery and relaxation. These things will make me stronger. I'll start so I can feel like I'm supporting myself.
I don't have the money.	I don't need extra money. I buy food anyway. I'll just make leaner choices. Leaner choices are cheaper. I'll actually save money without all the expensive processed foods with added sugar and fat.
I don't like dieting.	I don't have to feel like I'm dieting and being deprived. I can still have pleasure and enjoy wide varieties of food. In fact, I'll be eating better than I have in a long time. I'm going to enjoy this experience, I'm going to develop a new relationship with food.

I'm lazy, I admit it.	Nutrition and exercise is going to give me energy and a sense of well-being I haven't felt in a long time. I'll just start. I need a pick-me-up.
I was born to be fat.	I was born to be lean. This issue about fat might be less personal if I say *I have fat*, or I temporarily have fat, instead of *I am fat*. Fat isn't part of my identity. It's just something I have, and I can let it go.
I don't know how to do it.	I'll just start eating from the four food groups, and by a week or two, I'll be losing fat and I'll know how to do it.
I don't like exercise.	I love to feel the air on my skin during a walk outdoors. I like to feel my muscles getting strong while rowing. I love the feeling of exercise because it makes me feel young.

To develop affirmation, or positive-feedback to yourself, you also need a positive outlook on life. It's hard to have that if you are always criticizing yourself. Stop all criticism and begin to tell yourself only positive things. You can build up the strength you need to stay positive by beginning to practice behavior techniques like relaxation and deep breathing for stress control. You'd be surprised how strong they can make you feel in a very short time. Start your exercise program with walks, or one aerobic selection that pleases you. When it begins to bore you, switch to another. Increase your activity and exercise gradually as you get stronger and more nutritionally fit.

The simplest way to get the drop on your rationalizations is to start tomorrow by fixing your food day. That alone will give you unexpected energy, and you'll feel better about everything. *See* Food Groups.

● **RDAs** Recommended daily allowances for nutrients, vitamins and minerals based on your body's need for growth, repair, and maintenance (metabolism). Rather than worry, the best way to get them is to meet the serving requirements in the food group system on a daily basis. Only after that, should you consider eating other foods. *See* Food Groups.

▲ **REGAIN** A relapse following a diet, entering the yo-yo syndrome and gaining weight back. *See* Relapse. Yo-Yo Syndrome. Rapid Weight Loss.

▲ **RELAPSE** Weight regain immediately following a diet. This occurs more frequently after diets that are too low in calories, too restrictive, and used for rapid weight loss. It is particularly true of diets that remove carbohydrates, or use any form of imbalanced food plan. The major reason for regain after these types of diets isn't your eating habits, it's your metabolism and body composition. You're at ideal weight with a very low burning metabolism, caused by the dramatic calorie restriction. And you've lost muscle, which doesn't give you the body composition you need to keep fat away.

If you're coming off a plan that was very restrictive, and you're starting to regain, you have to stop the regain in the first stages. It will take a little work, but you can do it. The last thing you should do is go back on a low-calorie plan that is very restrictive. It will create the same problems, and you may not see weight loss at all. You have to retrain your body to burn more calories, and that means eating from all food groups, keeping your calories in a range that is more like the diet you should have tried in the first place. You need to exercise while you diet.

Food energy is the source to rebuild muscle protein you lost on the rapid diet, and the exercise keeps the process stabilized. Food kicks up your metabolism, especially in the proportions identified in the food groups, when you eat the leaner versions of those foods.

At first, you'll see some water weight and you have to get through that stage, but after a week or two, your body will start to stabilize, if you diligently replace your water, and eat a balanced diet. Use the plan to get yourself back to ideal weight, which needs to be slow, not rapid, to keep your metabolism at a higher burning level. When you get back to your ideal, remain on the diet for a week or two, until you are sure you've stabilized, then you can move on to maintenance.

This acts as a re-entry phase to help you repair the damage caused by losing weight too rapidly. Don't use this as permission to go on a rapid weight loss diet again, thinking you can pull yourself out again the next time. Each time you use rapid weight loss, your regain potential gets greater, and it's not healthy to keep throwing your metabolism out of sync. If you find yourself regaining again, go back to a full food diet at no less than 1000-1200 calories for women, no less than 1400-1600 calories for men, to bring yourself back into line. *See* Food Groups. Maintenance.

▲ **RELAXATION** A self-enriching skill. It's the backbone of success, used to renew you, beat stress, and drive you forward to success.

There are two basic approaches to relaxation.
BODY TO MIND — Using physical techniques to relax your body, which in turn, relaxes your mind. Examples are Deep Muscle Relaxation, Stretches, Callanetics, Yoga, Akido, Tai Chee, Massage, Diaphragm Breathing.
MIND TO BODY — Using mental techniques to relax your mind, which in turn relaxes your body. Examples are Deep Muscle Relaxation (mental), Meditation, Relaxation

Response, Bio-feedback, Hypnosis.

Both seek the same result: harmony of body/mind through release of tension. Since your body and mind are a team, it is difficult to separate one from the other in either process of relaxation, and the best programs include both aspects. For instance, in the body to mind program Callanetics, while you are using stretches to release your tension, the music creates a soothing mood, the voice is caring and comforting, and the lighting and visuals are not distracting. The result is a combined mind/body relaxation, or *deep muscle meditation.* This is an example of relaxation as an art.

However, it is possible to do one without achieving the other. You can use stretches for relaxation, and fail to quiet your stressed mind (mental resistance). Or you can use meditation, and fail to relax your stressed muscles (physical resistance). Your goal is to learn how to do *both* simultaneously. The art of relaxation is achieving it. Feeling it. One moment of release can compensate for hours, if not days, of stress.

The benefits of relaxation are also inter-related:

- Your pulse, heart rate, and respiratory rate decrease (relieving stress)
- Your breathing becomes more even and deeper (oxygen uptake is more effective)
- Your brain emits soothing alpha waves (wellbeing waves)
- Your blood lactate decreases (an ester of lactic acid, which is associated with neurosis)
- Your body is refreshed
- You are more receptive to learning in this state
- You are more capable of doing imagery or visualization in this state (claiming or owning a more positive future)
- Everything works better because you do.

THE RELAXATION INITIATOR

The first part of relaxation is the technique that sets the stage for fuller relaxation, and use of other skills. In a sense, it's like an enzyme — it catalyses other responses.

You can use this technique by itself or use it to initiate other, deeper suggestions.

Find a quite spot where you won't be disturbed. A soft, comfortable chair. Dim the lights. Sit straight but not tensed. Close your eyes and clear your mind. If your mind wanders, allow the thoughts to pass through, float them on a cloud.

Breathe in to the count of 3
one two three
Hold it lightly for the count of 3
four five six
Exhale to the count of 3
seven eight nine
As you exhale, let all of your muscles relax ...
Repeat
As you continue to breathe
deeply, let yourself go deeper
and deeper into relaxation ...

THE RELAXATION ADJUNCTS
(Choose one skill at each session to add on to the Relaxation Initiator)

DEEP MUSCLE RELAXATION

Starting with your toes, progressively relax each muscle group from your feet to your scalp. Feel relaxation spreading through your body. Use the feeling of heat or warmth to enhance the release "My toes are warm and limp...My feet are warm and limp"...Feel your muscles loosen up and expand. Continue to the top of your scalp.

FULL BODY RELEASE

Imagine your body as a sack of sand. Picture pin holes in the bottom of the bag. Sand is seeping out the holes. As the sand seeps out, you feel more and more relaxed. Picture a situation during the day which caused you tension. Let it flow out of the bag with the sand.

FINDING YOUR PERFECT PLACE
Visualizing Your Place

Find a scene from nature which gives you joy and pleasure. An ocean vista. A wheat field in the wind. A garden of flowers. Hills in Vermont. Put yourself in the picture. You are lean and light in this picture. Your weight doesn't go with you. Become part of the scene. Feel the air, the sun. Be there...If people or animals come into the place, wave to them and let them pass through. You own this place ...it's your space to be completely protected and safe...nothing can hurt you in this place...Smile at anything that arrives and wave goodbye to it...feel the air as you do it...inhale and exhale evenly. Relax and enjoy this place as long as you want to.

LATER: When something or someone stresses you, bring up the picture of this place...feel the air and comfort...breathe deeply...None of the stresses go with you into this place...they can't get in because the place won't let anything stress you...it's your perfect place.

Breathe in to the count of 3
one two three
Hold it lightly for the count of 3
four five six
Exhale to the count of 3
seven eight nine
As you exhale, let all of your muscles relax ...
Repeat
As you continue to breathe
deeply, let yourself go deeper
and deeper into relaxation ...

THE RELAXATION ADJUNCTS
(Choose one skill at each session to add on to the Relaxation Initiator)

VISUALIZATION FOR PROBLEM-SOLVING

Eating
Picture a situation where you are ready to eat something very fattening or very sweet. Then picture yourself not eating it, and laughing.

Stress
Picture yourself covered in a mountain of paper, stressed. Picture a wind coming in and blowing the paper away like day moths.

Stressors
Picture your boss stressed at you. Picture the stress falling off him/her like feathers. Picture him/her smiling and congratulating you.

Mental Rehearsal
Invent your own problem scene and resolve it. For instance, create a scene where you might eat and imagine yourself doing something else.

Exercise
Picture yourself lying on the couch too tired to move. Picture air coming in and lifting you up. Picture yourself walking, running, rowing or cycling and loving it.

Mental Rehearsal
Invent your own sedentary scene and resolve it.

IMAGERY ON PAPER

See Fear of Failure to learn how to draw positive imagery pictures to resolve negative emotions.

RISKS Conditions associated with excess weight. The more weight you gain, the greater the strain on your body system. Weight-related risks range from mild disorders to major diseases. This does not mean that an overweight person can't be free of disease or disorders. It means there is a greater tendency for these conditions to occur. If specific conditions are already present, excess weight can aggravate conditions. If family history shows a tendency toward a specific disease, excess weight can increase the likelihood of acquiring this disease.

Arrythmias
Arteriosclerosis
Blood Pressure
Cancer
Carcinoma
Cerebral Hemorrhage
Cirrhosis of Liver
Diabetes
Edema
Gallstones
Gout
Heart size-left ventricle
Hernias
Hypertension
Impotency
Inflammation of Veins
Insulin Levels
Lower Back Problems
Menstrual Irregularities
Orthopedic Problems
Osteoarthritis
Renal Disease
Rupture of Spinal Disks
Skin Irritations
Skin Ulcers
Stroke
Surgical Risks
Susceptibility to Infections
Triglyceride Levels
Venostasis
Yo-Yo Syndrome

Body Functions

Glucose Metabolism
Good Cholesterol
Insulin Sensitivity
Intestinal Motility
Mechanical Efficiency
Metabolic Function
Mobility
Sex Drive
Reproductive Capacity

Based on 40-90 pounds of excess weight.

● **ROUGHAGE** Fiber. *See* Fiber.

◆ **ROWING** Stationary aerobic exercise machine or outdoor aerobic sport.

Benefits:
- Excellent cardiovascular training.
- Great calorie-burning exercise.
- Works upper and lower body, improving strength and mobility.
- No orthopedic injury.
- Pace and tension are easily adjusted.
- Very portable; stores in small space.
- Can be used for additional strength building exercises.

Guidelines:
- Adjust the tension of the arm pulls to the lowest level.
- Sit on the seat cushion and strap feet into stirrups. Make sure handles of the rowing arms are parallel to your foot pads.
- Position the seat up to your feet so that you're in a crouched position. Keep your back straight and grasp the handles of the rowing arms.
- Glide the seat backward, straightening your legs, and pull the rowing arms until your legs are fully extended and your hands are parallel to your body. (For a full arm extension, bend your arms past your body and fully extend.)
- Return to starting position by gliding the seat forward, bending your knees and simultaneously pushing the rowing arms back to the start.
- The pace at which you row and the rowing arm tension determine the intensity of your workout. Start slow!
- Wear racquet gloves to prevent or minimize blisters. *See* Exercise.

S

▲ **SABOTEURS** Cues (people, situations, things) that cause you to feel less secure about success. A saboteur can be a person who tries to tempt you to break your diet, situations that lure you to eat excess food, or unexpected events that cause extra stress, and its effect, you think you might fail.

When you are on a diet, it can seem like everything and everyone is trying to subvert your success. A family member might say: "I liked you better when you weren't dieting." A friend might comment: "Go ahead and have dessert. I won't tell." Even though these people might not intend to subvert you, inadvertently they do. Events can compound your stress during a diet. For instance, the week you start dieting, you find out that your best friend is getting married and wants you in the wedding party. That means parties and food. Or work pressures increase, family crises develop, and that means added stress. It might seem that Murphy's Laws are running your life when you start a diet – "If things can go wrong, they will."

It's important to remember that any change in your life – such as a diet – will create its own set of problems in the first phases. After all, it's notice to people that *you intend to change,* and that upsets their old familiar routines with you. This can be particularly threatening to people who have centered their relationship with you around food, with you as the food preparer, or you as the companion for all-you-can-eat lunches. The key to solving these upsets is found in your attitude. You can face these issues as challenges to your *skillpower,* not threats to your *willpower.* When it comes to successful dieting, skill counts, not will. Skills are positive sets of solutions you can use to strengthen your resolve and make you self-sufficient. Learning to be assertive about your decision is an important skill. That means you can say "no thanks" to dessert, without getting angry at the person who is offering it. It means you can ask your best friend to include low-fat alternatives to the standard wedding buffet, without feeling embarrassed about speaking up for yourself. Remember who you are trying to change – YOU – not everyone else, and keep a sense of humor about their responses to your diet.

Use crisis situations as opportunities to learn how to gain control over your eating patterns and emotional habits, rather than triggers to let go. Review your goals each day, and reaffirm your commitment to succeed. Reinforce yourself daily with relaxation exercises for stress reduction and behavior techniques for positive self-support – skillpower! Keep a journal of problem situations that occur and the strategies you used to combat them. Review your journal regularly, adding new possibilities for creative solutions as you progress. Most of the behavior skills developed for successful dieting are strength-giving and will enrich your whole life. Each time you triumph over a difficult situation, congratulate yourself with a reward that isn't food, such as tickets to a play you've wanted to see, a walk with a close friend. Your goal on a diet is to become a successful problem-solver. Eventually, you won't have to keep a journal about problems and solutions, the solutions will snap into play when problems emerge, because they will be ingrained and natural. *See* Food Cues.

SACCHARIN A crystalline compound used as a sugar substitute, more than 300 times sweeter than sugar. Studies indicate it causes cancer. It has no energy value. No evidence suggests it aids in weight loss. *See* Artificial Sweeteners.

SAFE WEIGHT LOSS Removing fat from its stores, while providing the nutrition that's needed for muscle protection and health. Safe weight loss is generally regarded as losing 1.5% of your body weight per week. It means fat loss, not muscle losses. To accomplish this, the diet you choose must provide your essential daily nutrients. Without these nutrients, nothing works right. The preferred calorie level for women is 1000-1500 calories per day, but not below 1000. The preferred calorie level for men is 1400-1800, but not below 1400. The best choice is real food, not the processed variety with added sugars and salts (and fats). The program should fit into your lifestyle so you'll keep doing it. You should go for the maximum, not the minimum in variety, personal pleasure, and a positive diet experience. You should exercise simultaneously, which is why you need more energy calories from carbohydrates, which seldom store as fat. Your weight loss should be slow and steady to insure that you are only losing fat. You can see water fluctuations, but if you learn to gauge your weight loss *range,* instead of your weight loss each day, you won't be fooled by water changes. You must drink plenty of water while you are on a diet to facilitate all of the metabolic processes and mobilize your fat. And you should always take a vitamin/mineral supplement any time you diet, as a secondary support for nutrition.

The decade of the eighties was the age of the rapid weight loss diets. The lessons that were learned were based on failure. These lessons were: rigid calorie restriction, strict rules and deprivation, no-and low-carbohydrate menus, abnormal eating patterns, your foods and my foods — all of these techniques create rapid weight regain. *See* Food Groups for guidelines to evaluate or create a balanced food plan.

● **SALT** *See* Sodium.

SATIETY Nutrient satisfaction, or the *off* signal that follows hunger when it is abated. *See* Appetite.

SATURATED FAT. The fat in food that is considered poor fat, because it raises the level of LDL or bad cholesterol in your body. *See* Cholesterol.

◆ **SAUNA SUITS** Rubberized outfits promoted as "slimming" gear. The only thing they slim is your potential for healthy weight loss. These suits provide an artificial weight loss from water displacement. If you wear a sauna suit and exercise for 20 minutes, you'll feel perspiration dripping from your body, and you'll weigh less when you get on the scale. You're seeing temporary water losses, not fat losses, and you could be courting danger.

These suits should never be used in hot humid weather because they prevent your body from cooling naturally, by trapping perspiration next to your skin. For proper evaporation to occur, your skin needs to come into contact with a steady circulating stream of air, which rubberized suits prevent. In hot weather, these suits can cause heat stroke, heat exhaustion, chronic dehydration and even death. A better bet is to skip the suit and do the 20 minutes of exercise. That way, you get the benefits without the risks.

▲ **SCALE, BODY WEIGHT** A combination of your fat, muscle and water in pounds. Your scale tells you more about the flow of water in and out of your body than it does about fat. Water is approximately 60% of your body weight. When you are looking down at that number in the metal box, you could be reading water retention from too much salt. Or you could be reading water losses from an active exercise session on a hot day. The numbers can trick you into actions that might not be appropriate. For instance, if your scale reads that you lost three pounds of water, you might think you lost fat, so it's OK to have a dinner at your local restaurant (where you know they cook with fat). Or you might feel frustrated when your scale reads the same after a week of dieting, and you might stop. A day later, you lose the water that you were retaining and you see a sudden drop in weight (last night you quit your diet and ate everything in the refrigerator, because you were sure your diet wasn't working). Relying on your scale to measure your weight loss success is like asking a mirror in a fun house to tell you how you look tonight. The scale is responsible for more diet headaches than appetite suppressants on an empty stomach.

Rely on getting looser in your clothing and tightening your belt a notch, instead of standing on the scale every day.

If the scale were perfect, this is what it would look like:

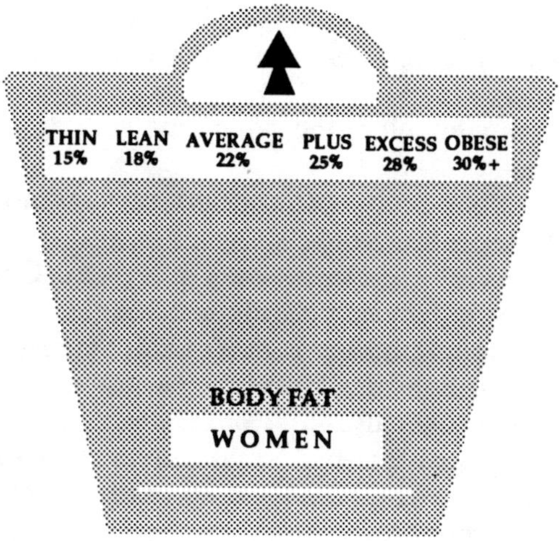

Based on underwater weighing of athletes.

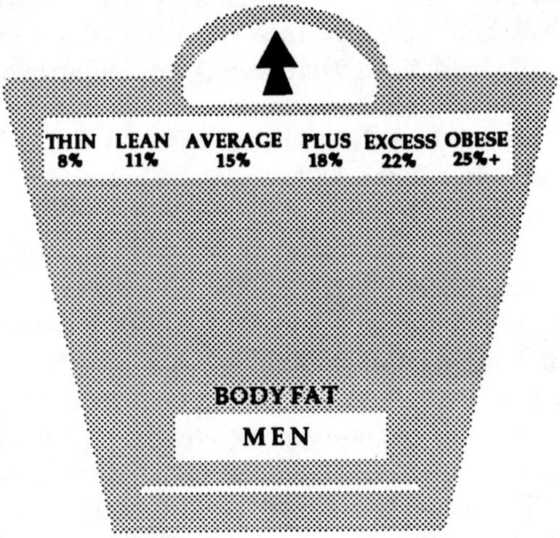

It would tell how much body fat is standing on the box. Then you could subtract that from 100%, and the rest would be your lean muscle.

Because the scale isn't an accurate indicator of your body composition, you have to outsmart it.

➡ How To Weigh Yourself

1. Weigh yourself before breakfast, after your bladder is emptied.
2. Weigh yourself at the same time very day, in the same way.
3. Wear light clothing (or underwear) and no shoes.
4. Add up your weekly weights and divide by 7 to determine your average weekly weight. Compare that average to the lowest and highest weight of the week for your average weight range. Your average weight range will tell you how much weight variation you can expect on a weekly basis (usually from water fluctuations).
5. The pounds lost below your average weekly weight are as close as you can come to reading your actual fat loss, using your scale.

If you are on a healthy diet that uses lean protein for muscle protection, low-fat for fat removal, and carbohydrates for energy — the actual weight loss will be fat loss.

If you are on a rapid weight loss diet that is very low calorie, you can see dramatic water losses and muscle losses, so there is no way for you to tell what's going on, when you stand on the scale.

If you are a woman, you have to take your monthly ovulation cycle into account, when you can see greater fluctuations in water weight.

If you are retaining too much water, diuretics are not the best choice. Reduce your salt intake and drink more water to bring yourself back into balance.

If you find that your clothing is looser, but the scale doesn't register any difference, don't despair. You could be increasing your muscle content and muscle is heavier than fat.

If you are starving yourself to lose weight, the losses you see on the scale are primarily muscle and water. You are going to make it easier to gain back your fat.

If you are watching the numbers go down slowly (say 2 pounds per week) and you are sticking to your diet, congratulations! You know how to play the numbers and win. You're losing your fat. The interesting thing about fat loss is how it appears on your body. **Five pounds of fat loss *looks like* ten pounds of weight loss** (which can be water, muscle and fat). That's the real benefit of aiming for fat loss with a healthy diet. You lose fat slower, but you look better faster. And you set yourself up for lean body maintenance for life.

▲ **SCALE, FOOD** A kitchen device to weigh your food to conform to serving sizes recommended by a diet.

You do not have to use a measuring scale for your food, if you are not on a diet that limits your food to the maximum. You can use average serving sizes indicated in the food groups. If you want to be sure you're not overdoing your protein, weigh your proteins for a week, and teach yourself how to calibrate portion sizes with your eye. Then re-test yourself every few weeks to see how good your eye is. If you eat more than your share of vegetables and fruits, it isn't going to pack on fat. In fact, it will help to keep you lean. Studies indicate that complex carbohydrate foods take so long to digest that extras don't store as fat. This is how athletes stay slim, when they seem to eat so much more than the average person. Their *extras* are complex carbohydrates. The foods to watch closely are the fats and oils and sweets. They're the ones that take you over your fat maximum and sugar maximum. They combine to store fat. Keep your fiber content high and limit the amount of processed foods you eat. Make sure you get your daily calcium from low-fat milk and dairy products. Your measuring scale should be the proportions of food you eat: 60% complex carbs/20% lean proteins, 20% fat. When you get it down to a routine, you get lean.

SCREENING Tests to determine if you are able to go on a particular diet program. Most of the diets that need medical screening are very strict diets with low-calorie formats. You should never embark on a diet like that without proper screening. Under 800 calories should always be monitored by a doctor, especially if the diet doesn't include enough carbohydrates. Balanced food diets(1000-1500 cals/day for women; 1400-1800 cals/day for men) don't require screening, because these are the same standards your doctor would ask you to adhere to for safe weight loss.

● **SEASONINGS** Taste enhancers for dieters. *See* Herbs & Spices, for the list.

▲ **SELF ESTEEM** A feeling of self worth. Lack of self-esteem is usually associated with the overweight state, especially in obesity. This may not have been a problem before weight gain, (or it's likely it was), but nevertheless, after weight is gained and held for long periods of time, your sense of self worth begins to be more closely linked to food issues and fat problems. This is a form of projecting emotions and feelings into food. Regardless of your self-esteem issues, it's vital to learn how to like yourself as you are, and as you begin dieting. The success of your diet and fitness efforts are strengthened by a sense of self worth at the outset. If you start with too many negative feelings about yourself, then weight loss is viewed as the miracle solution, and all you've done is transfer all of those emotions and feelings to being thin. This is a form of extreme thinking that will not serve you well during or after your diet.

It's important to realize that no one is immune to negative self-criticism, or low self opinions, even thin people. In fact, many thin people spend excessive energy finding fault with themselves. Their small pads of fat are as large to them as your weight is to you. The weight problem has to be put in perspective. It's a situation you can deal with, but it doesn't have to be your identity. You *have* fat, fat isn't your identity. Even if you think that fat is part of your identity, you can use Mirror Exercises and Relaxation exercises to let go of this misconception. Many people make the mistake of identifying with their fat. If you have a headache, you don't say: "I am a headache." And yet, the language of weight suggests that you're supposed to take fat on as an identity, and say "I am fat."

Perhaps our society won't change and thin will always be perceived as a sign of greater self-esteem. But thin isn't identity either. A thin person can have just as many identity issues as a fatter person. In the meantime, practice Relaxation and Mirror Exercises, and social pictures of self-worth will have less of a hold. In the end, what really counts is what you think of yourself. *See* Relaxation. Mirror Exercises. Imagery.

ALL BEHAVIOR TOPICS BUILD SELF ESTEEM. *See* ▲

▲ **SELF IMAGE** How you see yourself from inside, regardless of the view from the mirror. *See* Mirror Exercises.

SERVINGS Standard measurements for food portions based on nutrient value and healthy eating (to stay lean). The food group system sets the requirements for standard servings, based on the needs of your metabolism to maintain your body, repair its cells, and facilitate all processes. These serving recommendations are the ones that are used for most eating plans and healthy diet programs across the country. However it is important to note that the meat group serving size has gotten a bit out of line, even in diet books and calorie counters. Most people think that a standard serving of meat is 4-6 ounces, when it really should be 2 ounces. This mistake can add a great deal of excess fat. The food industry isn't consistent with servings, and a TV dinner might have 4-6 ounces of meat. The labels usually have the correct serving size per total weight of the product, but it's best to check to be safe.

Your carbohydrate servings (complex carbohydrates) do not have to be as carefully watched as your protein and fat servings, because protein and fat add the most fat to your body, and the carbohydrates tend to burn off. Carbohydrates also have fiber which helps to prevent fat storage. This only refers to the natural carbohydrates such as fruits, vegetables and whole grains, since the processed varieties contain fats, sugars, salt and very little fiber.

It's a good idea to learn the standard servings, even memorize them. That way, you can be sure you're getting accurate information. A serving size mistake can cost you a lot of fat. For instance, you might read a calorie counter that gives the fat content of a candy bar, but it's a one ounce serving, while the standard candy bar is 2 ounces. In addition, most diet programs adapt the serving sizes to their overall calorie level, so that their serving size may be different from the required one. Because of all the variations in sources, few people know what the accurate requirements are. *See* Food Groups, for serving sizes.

SETPOINT A theory about metabolism that was popular in the '80s. An idea, rather than a scientific fact. The setpoint idea claimed that your body has an inner thermostat determined to keep you fat, or a weight you will return to despite a diet. This theory sprang out of research on the failure rates of diets, specifically rapid weight loss diets, which are notorious for causing rapid weight regain. It's a result of *poor* dieting that was taken out of context and sold as a fact of life.

If you think about a thermostat, you'll see the flaw in reasoning for setpoint. A thermostat only reads what is happening, it can't read what can happen. The thermostat in your car reads the existing heat level. If you stop the car and restart it later the thermostat will read that your car engine is cooler. The same thing applies to your metabolism. Your metabolic rate (thermostat) only reflects what you give it to work with. When you lose weight rapidly, your metabolic rate is reduced from calorie restriction and muscle losses. It reads cool. When you eat less fat, more fiber and adequate protein, you generate more metabolic heat from eating, even on a diet. The thermostat reads warm. When you exercise, you raise the heat production in your body by 15%, and the output continues after the exercise is over. Your metabolism is never set, or static. The combination of exercise and a heat-producing diet can drive up your metabolism to burn fat and build muscle, and that prevents weight regain. The thermostat reads *hot*.

● **SIMPLE SUGARS** Naturally-occurring sugars in carbohydrate foods. *See* Sugar. Carbohydrates.

◆ **SKIING** Skill sport aerobic exercise. *See* Exercise.

◆ **SKILL SPORTS** Aerobic exercises including tennis, racquetball, squash, handball, skiing, basketball, volleyball, and so forth.

Benefits:
- Easily combined with a more regular aerobic routine.
- Add variety and excitement, challenging a partner or joining forces with a team.
- Considered play rather than workout.

Guidelines:
- Play as frequently as possible to improve skill, since skill level determines intensity.
- Couple these games with other aerobic activities to equal half an hour at least 3 times per week.
- Try to stay in continuous motion and minimize non-active time.

SKIN FOLD CALIPERS The metal instrument that resembles a giant tweezer used in anthropometric tests for body fat and muscle composition. *See* Anthropometric Measurements.

● **SNACKS** Energy boosters between meals. This can be a habit that adds a lot of sugar and fat if you choose low-nutrition snacks. But if you eat most of your snacks in complex carbohydrates — vegetables, fruits, whole grains — you'll have less hunger as a result. Complex carbohydrates are natural appetite suppressants.

THE BEST SNACK — any fruit, vegetable, whole grain. You can find many snacks that give you pleasure and don't add fat. This is particularly important to a dieter, who tends to think of restricted calories as a dreadful situation. It doesn't have to be that way.

If you rate your snacks for their fat content, it will provide an easy method to keep your fat moderated. The average lean snack should be 1-2 grams of fat.

Safe Sweet Treats and Snacks

Toast with Apple Butter and Cinnamon	1 Gram fat
Frozen Grapes	No fat
Jams, Jellies	No fat
Popcorn Plain	No fat
Angel Food Cake	No fat
Sugar Free Candies	No fat
Vanilla Wafer	1/2 Gram fat
Fig Bar	1/2 Gram Fat
Ginger Snap	1/2 Gram fat
Mini Chocolate Mint Patty	1 Gram fat
Yogurt Ice Cream	Low fat
Popsicle	No fat
Bread Sticks	No fat
Toast with Jelly	1 Gram fat
Any Fruit (except avocado, coconut)	No fat
Any Vegetable with No-fat Dip	No fat
A Cup of Pasta Salad with Vegetables (No-Fat Dressing)	2 Grams fat

There are numerous possibilities for non-fattening snacks that can make your dieting experience a pleasure. You do not have to starve yourself or deprive yourself of all pleasure to get slim. All you have to do is change habits like your high-fat snacking to lean snacking techniques. You can be satisfied on a diet and still burn fat.

● **SODAS (DIET)** Drinks with artificial sugar are usually considered dieter's sodas, but they shouldn't be. They have no nutritional value, and are simply sugar drinks with additives, even when they are low calorie. When you're on a diet, you want to get the most nutrition for your calories, and artificial sugars have no value. The long-term effects of artificial sweeteners have led to warnings about saccharin and have banned cyclamates, and the newest one, aspartame, is still being tested. Many dieters drink sodas by the six pack, thinking they're an acceptable way to ward off hunger. But they're not. Studies indicate that sweet drinks lead to an increased tolerance for sugar. If you're drinking sodas with artificial sweeteners, all you are getting is sweetness in a condensed form. This can make you want and need more sweets to be satisfied. Evidence shows that artificial sweeteners have no benefit for weight control.

What's the real diet soda? Club soda spritzers (lime, lemon, cranberry). Water plain or fruited. Fresh fruit juices for super nutrition. Cold herb teas provide an interesting change of pace. Low-fat milk is excellent and essential. Start limiting your use of diet sodas and turn to the drinks that give you greater nutrient density. That way, you get better fat burn and health.

● **SODIUM** Naturally-occurring mineral. Also called salt. In your body, sodium is found in body fluids and bones — 50% in your extracellular fluid, arteries, veins, capillaries, intestinal fluids, around your cells, and 50% in your bones.

In your diet, you get sodium in five ways:

- occurring naturally in foods (best source)
- added during processing (worst source)
- added during cooking (habit to limit)
- added at the table (habit to eliminate)
- from medications (source to control, where possible)

DON'T FORGET THAT
SODIUM & POTASSIUM
NEED TO BE BALANCED
SEE POTASSIUM

SODIUM IN BALANCE 1100 — 3300 mg per day	SODIUM TO EXCESS 3300 — 6000+ per day
It works with potassium to balance blood acid/alkali content.	Causes losses of potassium which create fluid retention, swelling and dizziness.
It helps to regulate fluid balance on both sides of cell walls.	Causes high blood pressure which leads to heart attacks and strokes
It's vital to muscle contraction/expansion.	Leads to kidney disease
It's vital for nerve stimulation.	
It keeps minerals soluble so they don't form deposits in your bloodstream.	
With Chlorine, it purifies your body of carbon dioxide, and aids digestion.	
It maintains blood volume and pressure by attracting and holding water in blood vessels.	

Sodium excesses are extensive in our modern-age microwave and TV dinner diets. It's second to sugar in additives used in processed foods as a preservative and flavor enhancer. Most of us are getting double the recommended daily dose, primarily from table salt misuse, cooking abuse and reliance on processed foods as a diet staple.

If you diet with fresh food sources as your primary foods, and use a pinch of sodium instead of a pour from the salt shaker, in cooking and at the table, you won't find sodium excesses in your diet. It's the easiest way to take control over sodium without doing endless calculations. And you gain another benefit from fresh foods — better fat burn and health.

If you are on a low-or-no sodium plan for your heart, use an herb salter to replace your regular salt for eating and cooking needs, and eliminate sodium-rich processed foods from your diet. Check our sodium-at-a-glance guide to find the foods highest in sodium, and beware that they don't sneak into your menus. Rely on natural foods, avoiding processed cheese foods and cured meats.

Shaking Off The Salt Habit. Sodium is a habit that is learned. Over time, as you increase the level of sodium in your food, you increase your taste for it. This process can easily be reversed by gradually reducing your sodium intake, thereby reducing your taste and desire for it. Many people find that it's better to go all out against sodium, enduring a saltless week or two, because it purifies your system and palate for salt, and you will immediately find salty foods undesirable, with your own taste buds acting as a regulator. Every so often, compute an average day's use of sodium to see if you're keeping within your limits. Sodium, like fat, has a tendency to sneak in, when you let down your guard.

Shopping Low Sodium

- Read labels for sodium content. Look for the exact content in milligrams. The label can say lower sodium and mean lower than the former version of that food.
- If sodium is not listed in milligrams, remember that label ingredients are listed first to last by weight. Sodium should be very low on the list, for safety.
- Learn to recognize high-sodium ingredients that can be listed on labels without saying sodium — such as baking soda, baking powder.
- Don't buy foods that don't have the sodium content listed. They aren't worth your trust.
- Don't forget to check labels on medications for sodium.

Diet/Sodium Sense

- Eat fresh foods whenever possible.
- Cut salt in your recipes to 1/2 or less.
- Replace high-sodium condiments with low sodium versions.
- Replace your salt with an herbal shaker for seasoning* in cooking and salting at the table.
- Taste your food before salting.
- In restaurants, ask for your food to be prepared salt-free.
- Ask for sauces and salad dressings on the side, so you can control the amount you use.

**Herb And Spice Salter*

You can make your own salt replacer that has no sodium. Mix your favorite herbs and spices to taste. Suggestions: onion powder, garlic powder, paprika, lemon peels, celery powder, red pepper and other spices of your choice. Experiment with blends until you achieve the perfect mix. Use it for cooking and table salting. No salt doesn't have to mean no taste.

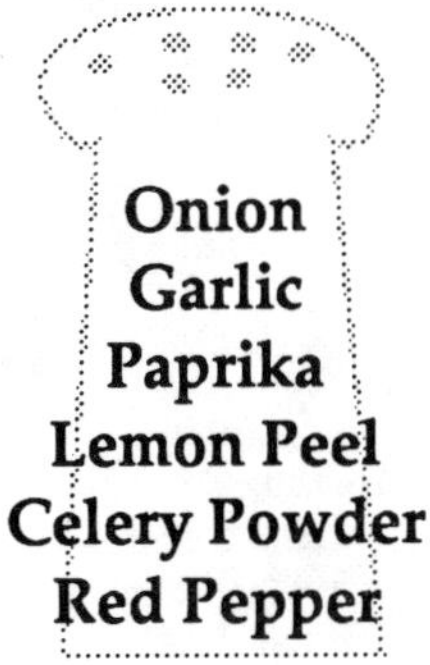

SODIUM AT A GLANCE
SOURCES OF EXCESS

Average Intake
2300-6900 mg/day

ELIMINATE OR MODERATE SOURCES OF EXCESS SODIUM

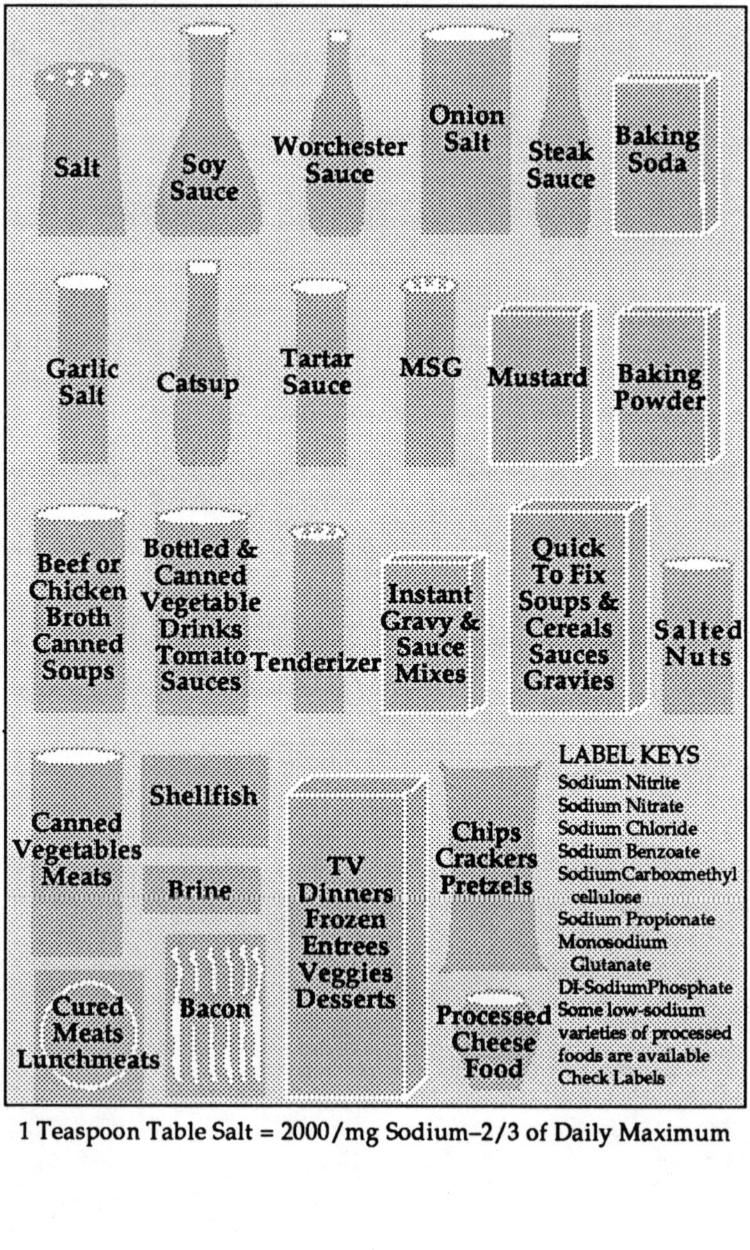

1 Teaspoon Table Salt = 2000/mg Sodium–2/3 of Daily Maximum

❤ BEST REPLACEMENTS

Recommended Dose
1100-3300 mg/day

RELY ON SODIUM THAT OCCURS NATURALLY IN FOOD

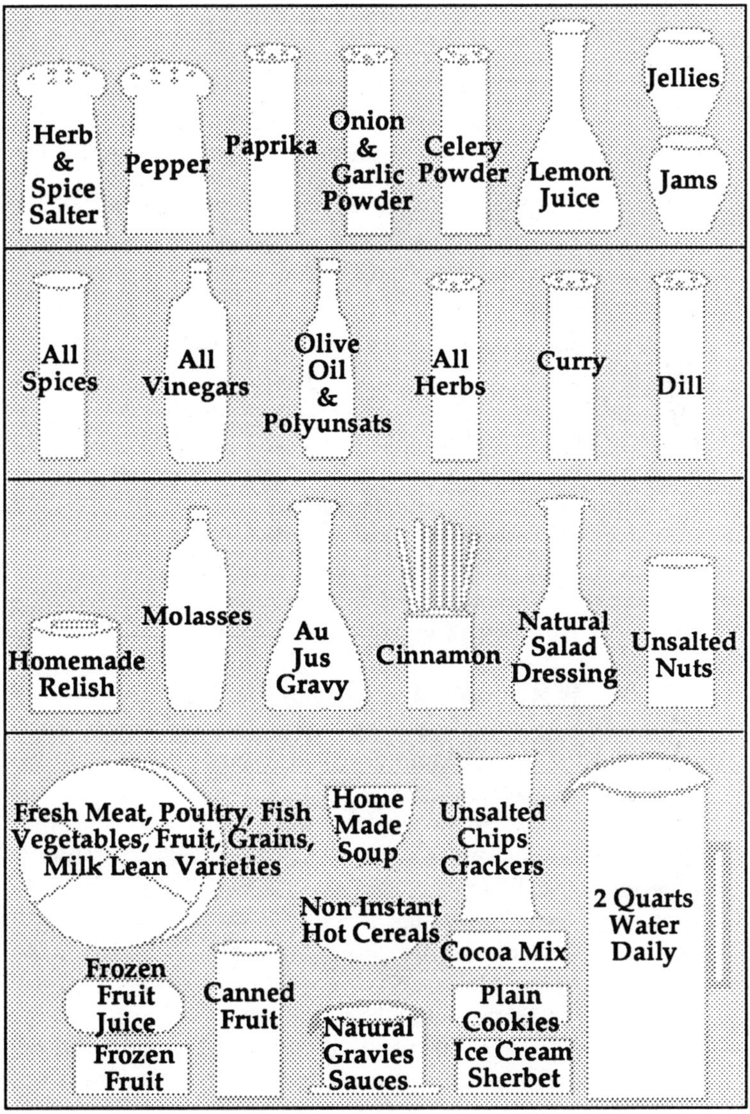

2 Teaspoon Herb & Spice Salter=0 mg Sodium=More Sodium Options

● **SOY** Vegetable protein. Nature's protein. Soy is a major source of protein for weight conscious dieters who are looking for a replacement for red meats or animal sources. Even though soy is listed as a grain, it is best to view it as a protein food, since it is the only natural grain that has about 10 grams of fat in a cup. When compared to an equivalent *protein,* soy is very low-fat. When you use it as a grain source, be aware that it's fatter than other grains, but it's still a remarkable food. Consider these important ingredients in soy:

High protein
Unsaturated fat
Low sodium
High fiber
Rich source of B complex, calcium, phosphorus, potassium, magnesium, iron, lecithin

❤ Lecithin in soy helps reduce cholesterol buildup by keeping cholesterol/calcium deposits in suspension. This prevents the deposits from adhering to artery walls.

Soy milk is a low-fat substitute for people who have allergies to regular milk. Soy oil is a good source of linoleic acid. Soy flour has a nutty taste for breads, gravies and sauces. Soybeans take a little time to soak overnight and cook. But they're worth it. *See* Grains.

SPARE TIRE Midriff weight, common to men. Men are primarily upper body fat distributors, depositing their fat in the midriff, chest and neck. This weight is easier to lose than lower body fat, but it's medically more risky, since it has been linked to heart disease. Weight lifting doesn't remove this fat, unless your diet is adjusted to remove fat in your food. Men get more of their fat from high-fat proteins, particularly steaks and red meats. The best plan is to switch to the leaner proteins such as chicken, turkey and fish, using the red meats less frequently, and choosing the lean ones. Fiber increases are important too, since fiber aids in fat loss and reduces the levels of bad cholesterol in your system – a heart saver. Men lose weight faster because of their greater percentage of muscle tissue, so a low-fat, high-carbohydrate, lean protein diet will flatten that tire. Women can be upper body fat distributors too, but they tend to get more of their fat from gravies, sauces and sweets. Removing these excesses and improving your overall diet, along with exercise will trim that tire in and give you back your hourglass curves.

● **SPICES** Seasonings and taste enhancers for dieters. *See* Herbs & Spices for the list.

◆ **STAIRMASTER** Stationary aerobic exercise machine. *See* Exercise.

STARCH BLOCKERS A fad of the '80s which consisted of a protein extracted from kidney beans. Chemical tests indicated that this form of protein blocked starch digestion by inhibiting the enzyme amylase (the enzyme in saliva that begins to break down carbohydrates). Supposedly, this caused starch (from carbohydrate foods) to pass into your intestines undigested like fiber, instead of being converted to glucose for absorption by your blood. However, human studies didn't show the same results as chemical studies. In humans, starch blockage was only about 10% of the total starch in the diet. It seems that the blockers couldn't hold their own when they met gastric juices and the acid composition of the stomach. Even if they worked, starch blockers would hardly be useful to a dieter, since starch in complex carbohydrates is one of the least fattening sources of energy. Remember, the starches are lean, calorie-burning foods, but the fats you put in them aren't. Your body requires starch for metabolism, and blocking can cause nutrient imbalance and digestive disorders. When starch breakdown is inhibited, your body uses protein and fat, and your metabolism can be distorted. The FDA put a halt to the sale of starch blockers for safety reasons, but a number of people paid the price in fat gain. Because they thought starch was not digesting, they ate more of everything, and gained weight.

It's never wise to interfere with the natural processes of metabolism, which require the nutrients in carbohydrates, protein and fat to function properly. You also need vitamins, minerals and water on a daily basis. This not only protects your health, but it also gives you the best fat burn. *See* Food Groups.

STARVATION (TOTAL FASTING) Chronic nutrient deficiency that causes severe metabolic stress. When you go without food for one day, your body's glycogen storage is used up. (Glycogen is the name for stored glucose, derived from carbohydrates in digestion). But your brain *needs* glucose for its energy and maintenance. With no glucose or glycogen stores, your body has to steal protein from its own cells, in order to make glucose (glucogenesis). At this point, starvation causes a gradual depletion of body parts, called muscle wasting. After a few weeks of starvation, your brain adapts, and can then use fat as a fuel (ketones from fatty acid breakdown). This temporarily stops the breakdown of body protein for fuel. After your fat stores are depleted, there's no where else to turn for energy, and your body uses its remaining protein for all of its fuel needs. If food is not introduced, drastic muscle losses occur and death follows.

If food is introduced, it takes months of nutrient therapy to rebuild body protein, and it's seldom rebuilt fully unless exercise is included, along with a low-fat diet. Often, metabolic and psychological changes can occur, which were not present before starvation.

How does this relate to a diet? Many diets use a mild form of starvation to achieve weight loss. While the results are not as extreme, the process is similar. Many dieters stop eating for a few days at a time, thinking they can take off weight fast. It's the worst thing you can do for your health. It only takes a day of starvation for your body to begin to steal its own protein. And that means less muscle, which in turn, leads to poorer calorie burn.

STIMULANTS Chemicals or substances that rev up your nervous system. *See* Appetite Suppressants. Caffeine.

STOMACH One of the primary organs of digestion. Your stomach breaks down food into smaller units to prepare them for the small intestines where digestion continues, and absorption of the nutrients takes place. Your stomach is J shaped and muscular with three areas that perform specific functions. The upper part acts as a storage center for food while digestion takes place in the middle and lower part. The upper part continues the breakdown of carbohydrates that began in the mouth with an enzyme from your salivary glands. The mid-part is where primary breakdown of proteins take place, and the lower part has a pump-like muscle action to move food into your small intestines. It takes from 4 to 7 hours for food to pass through your stomach. *See* Digestion.

STOMACH STAPLING Surgery for serious obesity problems. Part of the stomach is sealed off, to make the stomach capacity smaller. This prevents intake of excess food, because fullness occurs sooner.

▲ STRESS A high-tension system, speeded up. Also called the fight or flight response because that's the way you feel when you're under stress, like you want to run or fight, and most of the time, you can't do either one. Stress is a series of physiological changes that can be brought on by shock, change, or threat in your environment, or the perception of it in your mind. When stress occurs, you pump more adrenaline, your heart beats faster, your breath is short and shallow, your blood pressure is elevated, and blood rushes to your muscles (to run). Your blood vessels constrict to keep your system pressure up (to fight).

In emergency situations, stress can save your life. You can respond quicker, move faster, lift more weight, do things you thought you were afraid of. Some stress is necessary for growth and change, to motivate you to seek new challenges, set new goals, start new businesses, feel excited by life, reach optimal levels of performance in sports. Athletes face stress regularly, but it's considered good stress, because it has a physical outlet.

In non-emergency situations in daily life, stress often has no outlet. A traffic jam every morning, money constraints, time deadlines, job pressures, a sudden family crisis, any major change, threats to your security — all of these conditions bring on stress. Any situation which requires you to alter your behavior is stress producing. Your thoughts and feelings can exacerbate stress. Nutrient depletion puts you in a defenseless position against stress.

Dieters have to face two levels of stress — the normal, everyday stress that everyone else is facing, and stress peculiar to dieting.

Calories And Stress. Calorie reduction is stress. Your system adapts to using a certain calorie level for metabolism, and a sudden calorie decrease upsets the status quo. Your body has to work harder for its energy. If your diet doesn't provide the nutrients you need to meet that stress biochemically, your metabolism has to work at a deficit. It's one reason deprived diets are so dangerous for a dieter — metabolic stress.

Daily stress also depletes your nutrients. When your heart beats faster, and blood pressure rises, so does your metabolism. It burns nutrients faster. You have to replace the nutrients in your daily diet, or your body will take them from your muscles and bones. Daily nutrient insurance is a must for anyone facing stress, but particularly for a dieter.

Behavior and Stress. Dieting means changing your standard eating patterns into different ones. Change causes stress, even when the change is for the better. That's why it's important to choose a diet that uses natural eating patterns in a low-calorie format, instead of an un-natural diet that causes a great disruption in your lifestyle. The more unnatural the diet, the greater the stress to adhere to it.

Food and Stress. Stress leads to eating, particularly for a person who uses food for rewards or consolation. The more stressful your diet program, the greater the likelihood that you will eat to compensate for the feeling of deprivation and isolation from the world of food. That's why real food programs are better for you than low or no food programs with food substitutes. They create less food stress. Some programs say that removing people from food helps them resist food cues, and this allows greater weight loss. It also allows greater weight regain. The shock of re-entry into the world of food after months of deprivation is too stressful. You can't learn about eating and dealing with food by removing yourself from it. And you can't find good food habits in a pre-packaged box that says "one dinner." You have to use food to practice. You learn by doing, then repeating it until it becomes a habit.

Body Image and Stress. An image change occurs during dieting, and even when it's desired, it can be stressful. When you lose weight too fast, your image changes rapidly. In a sense, it runs ahead of you, and you're left with a thinner body that looks like it belongs to someone else. Rapid weight loss can disrupt your sense of self, and create image disturbances that leave you insecure about the results. This creates a great deal of emotional stress.

Your goal at the end of a diet is too important to be taken lightly. You shouldn't be scared out of your fat. You should move toward your thinner image gradually, using all the self-strengthening you can get to make the experience *feel* valid. Slow, steady change is far more genuine, and more supportive for long-term personal security. Often dieters set weight loss as their only goal, forgetting that there's a person on the diet, and that person needs to let go of their inner sense of weight, along with their outer one. When you get to ideal weight on strength instead of stress, that creates image balance, not disturbance.

Your World Vs. The World. The diet you choose should help you cope with the world of food opportunities, not remove you from them. When you choose deprived diets with special foods, you won't be able to find those foods in your supermarket. You can't adapt those foods to your ethnic background. If you have a family, you have to cook one thing for them, and have another food for you. Your food won't be found in restaurants, in vacation spots, and at family gatherings. You've got to carry a lunch box through life. This creates stress every time you face a vacation, party, or restaurant. You might stop going out for the duration of your diet, because these situations are too threatening. Diet isolation is an extreme form of stress. The solution isn't found by compounding your sense of separation. The solution is to form a new relationship with food.

Suddenly/Maintenance Stress. The more natural your diet, the easier it will be to shift into weight maintenance. The more abnormal your diet, the greater the gap between weight loss and maintenance. You can fall into that gap between your diet pattern and a lifestyle pattern and stay there for a long time, when you diet too differently from everyday life. If you spend a few months eating oddly on a diet, you've ingrained odd eating habits, and they are hard to shake. How do you go home and suddenly eat and live creatively with your thinner body? You don't.

You go home and eat to compensate for eating oddly for several months.

When your diet eating plan is too different from normal eating plans, it cannot be fixed by a six week maintenance program that tries to jam in all the things that make a positive lean life. It's too late by then. You have to start all over again, or face months of re-entry. This creates stress at ideal weight, when the stress should be abating. A balanced food diet is the best for maintenance program, because it's a dress rehearsal for the way you will live for life at higher calories. The food skills you learn during dieting carry over to maintenance, and you can eat more calories with an awareness of food content, sources of better food energy, and how to use food as your friend, not your enemy.

THE BEST DIET FOR STRESS DEFENSE

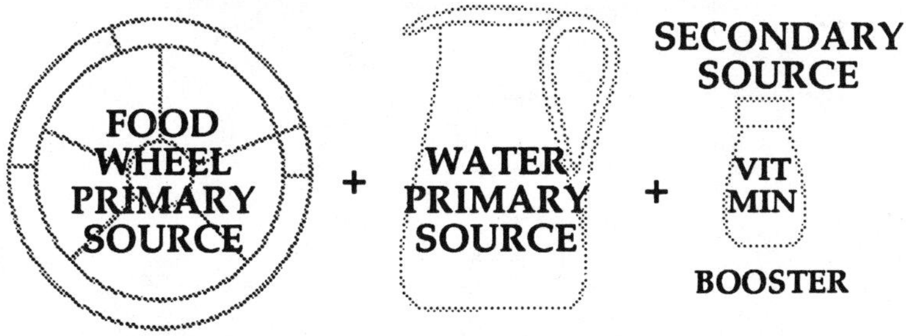

Minimizing diet stress is essential, since stress has been linked to most of the major lifestyle diseases including hypertension, heart disease and cancer. Stress reduction techniques like relaxation, meditation and deep breathing exercises are as important as nutritious food. They recharge your mind, attitude, perceptions and belief systems. Not only do they make your diet experience less stressful, they're tools to use in other areas of your life.

If you think about stress and the fight or flight feeling it gives you, you have two choices to make. You can run from it or fight. If you stand there and take it, stress will get the best of you. The best way to fight stress is to build a defense or shield. The next page shows you how.

Creating Your Lifestyle Shield. If you face stress without defenses like nutrition, exercise, relaxation, and personal pleasures for yourself, you'll have to take flight, because your system isn't built up to handle stress.

But when you create a lifestyle shield for yourself, using a regular routine for self-enhancement, you can face stress like a warrior. When you learn these skills for dieting, you've got them on your side for life. It's a life defense for stress.

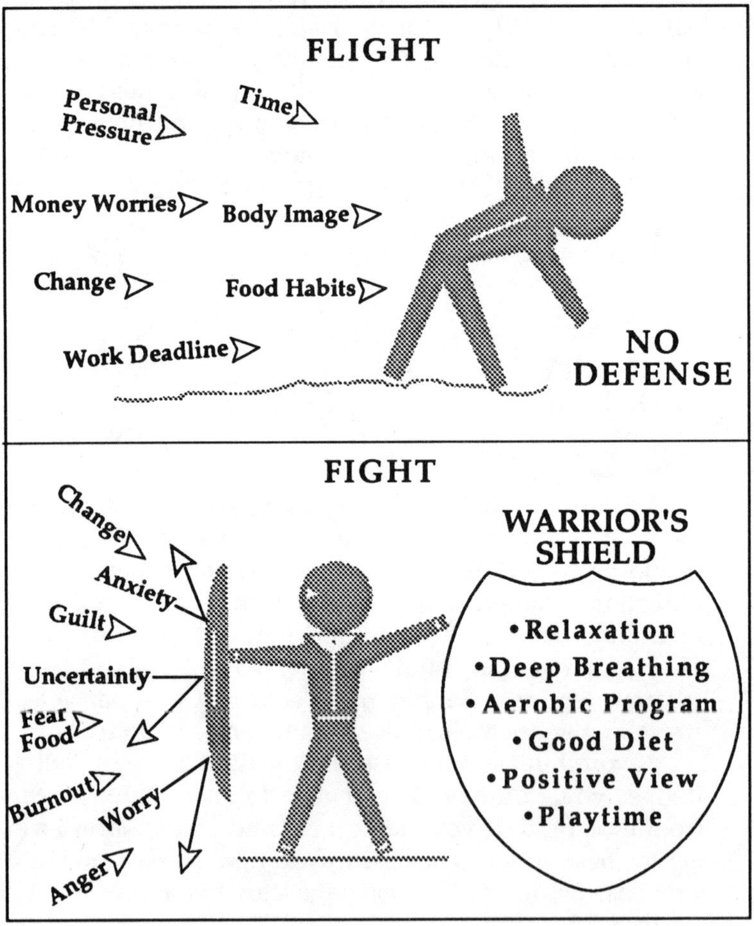

◆ **STRETCHING** Exercises to lengthen or elongate muscles and spine, loosen joints and increase overall co-ordination. Stretches are usually combined with breathing exercises for the best oxygen uptake. The effect of stretching is excellent for total body energy and grace. Excellent start up exercises for obesity.

▲ **SUBLIMINALS** Audio or visual tapes that contain underlying messages for unconscious teaching or training. Self-help tapes. Subliminal tapes usually contain affirmation messages under pictures, music or talk, but it is a good idea to be sure the messages are positive. The best choice is one that allows you to turn up the volume and hear the message, or turn up your TV screen to see the message. Written scripts aren't suitable, since a script is a separate entity. Subliminals have been used for relaxation training, stop-smoking programs, and motivational training in many areas. Subliminals are based on studies of the unconscious, where perception and learning is different from the normal waking state. Sleep learning is a part of this category, but most subliminals available on the market are not sleep training tapes. Those that can put you to sleep usually indicate that they are not to be used while driving or doing other active work.

Subliminal tapes can be helpful as an adjunct to diet and exercise, but it's not a good idea to rely on them as a solution. There is evidence that this form of training is easily forgotten, and therefore, must be repeated regularly. Anything positive is a good support aid, but it might be better to train yourself in positive thinking and affirmations on a more conscious level. That way, you're making a conscious choice to make positive changes, and you can enjoy the process of self-awareness that is associated with conscious choice. For instance, when you change negative statements you make about yourself to positive ones, in a conscious way, you can feel the effect on your system, and you can notice some interesting things about yourself. What you think, how you react, how you talk back to yourself, all of these responses lead to self-awareness. If you leave that process to a subliminal tape, it's not your voice and your process, and the effect is less permanent. The best plan would be to combine both.

▲ **SUBSTITUTION BEHAVIORS** Habits replaced for other habits, such as substituting exercise or relaxation exercises for eating binges. Substitution behaviors are the basis of behavior modification for weight loss and positive lifestyle change. *See Lifestyle,* for an easy way to use this powerful technique.

▲ **SUCCESS** Goal achievement. Successful dieting is viewed differently by the scientific community and dieters themselves. In science, success means maintaining your weight loss for at least two years after dieting. This is called medically significant weight loss. To the average dieter, success means losing weight (preferably as soon as possible). This is a very important issue because it influences the diet you choose. If you expect success to be weight loss only, you can probably achieve your goal on a number of diets, even poor ones that allow you to lose body muscle. But you can't expect to maintain your weight loss unless you choose a balanced diet that includes exercise, habit change, nutrition education, food cue control and self-strengthening components. These fall into the category of lifestyle diets.

The least promising diets for weight loss and maintenance are rapid weight loss diets, since regain is highest in this diet group. Despite this fact, dieters buy into them again and again repeating patterns of failure that are physically harmful and emotionally draining. Dieters are left feeling there is something wrong with them, when there is something wrong with the diet. Once of science's goals is to make people realize that slower weight loss is ideal weight loss. But this is hard to do in a fast-paced society where everything is expected A.S.A.P.

The best course for you is to re-define your expectations, to want more out of a diet than short-term slimness, because it's painful to get there after a lot of hard work, only to find you're losing the one thing you really wanted – staying there and enjoying the fruits of your efforts. In addition, you don't want to repeat failure too often, as you can with rapid weight loss diets, because failure can become ingrained like a habit on automatic pilot, and fear of failure can inhibit other decisions you make in your life. Keep in mind that dieting is something you are doing *for* yourself, not *to* yourself. The more skills you gain during your diet phase, the better equipped you will be to sail through maintenance and celebrate your life.

SUCCESS KEYS

When you are planning to lose weight, you are standing in front of three doors. One door is Diet, one is Exercise, and one is Behavior — you in the diet. Many programs are like the TV show "The Price Is Right." You only get to choose one door. When you do that, you can lose the big prize. That's a gamble you shouldn't take with your body. You need the keys to open all three doors, and success is yours.

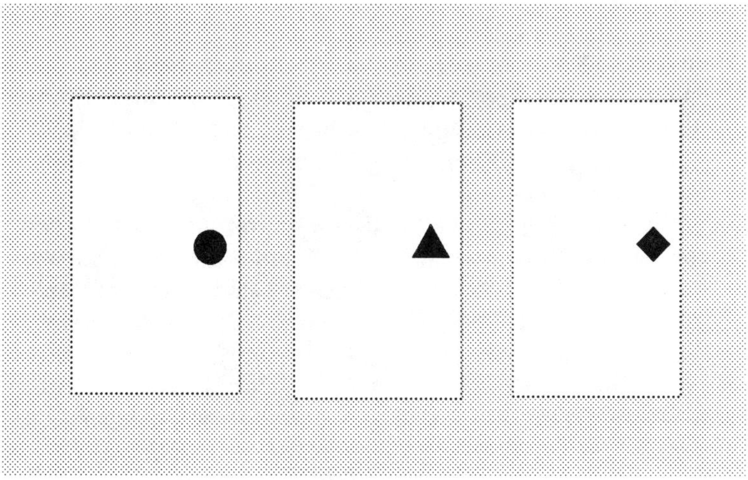

● Food Skills ▲ Behavior Skills ◆ Exercise Skills

● **SUGAR** A sweet tasting, water-soluble carbohydrate. There are three ways you get sugar in your food, but only one way to insure that you're not getting the *empty calorie* version of sugar.

All Natural Sugar. This is sugar that is an indigenous part of a food, such as sugar in an orange or apple. In this form, sugar is a naturally-occurring carbohydrate in low-fat format that provides vitamins, minerals, essential nutrients and fiber. Perfect diet food. The calories are packed with nutrition and metabolic clout.

Refined sugar. This is sugar removed from its source food, increased in potency and used as a garnish or ingredient in processing. Table sugar is double barrelled sucrose — 1/2 fructose and 1/2 dextrose. Corn syrups are also refined, and combine high-fructose and dextrose. Refined sugars can be the entire calorie content of a food or beverage, such as jelly beans or cola, which are 100% sugar. These varieties of sugars are the ones that give sugar its empty calorie reputation, not the naturally-occurring ones. Stripped from its source food, sugar has no vitamins, minerals, or nutrient benefits, even though it is still energy.

Processed Foods with Refined Sugars Added. These are the foods that spell trouble for dieters. The sugar isn't the biggest problem, even though processed foods typically have sugar-to-excess. The problem is *all* of the ingredients taken together — they add up to fat.

Take a look at the following comparison between a fresh food carbohydrate (pasta salad with vegetables) and a processed imitator (boxed pasta salad with vegetables). The fresh food version is a natural complex carbohydrate made with fresh-cut vegetables and any plain pasta, garnished with a no-fat, spicey salad dressing (genuine carbohydrate). The imitator is a pre-mixed pasta salad in a box.

WHAT DEFINES A CARBOHYDRATE FOOD?	
GENUINE CARBOHYDRATE	**CARBOHYDRATE IMITATOR (PROCESSED)**
Fiber content is high	Fiber is stripped out
Fat content is low	Fat is added in (sauce)
Simple sugar occurs	Double barrelled sugar added
High Vitamin/Mineral content	Nutrition stripped out
Protein (when it occurs is intact)	Protein damaged in processing
Chewability (Activates digestion)	Smooth and easy to swallow
Low calorie overall	High calorie

You decide. Do processed carbohydrate foods look like the real thing to you? A decade of confusion and misinformation has centered around carbohydrates. Dieters learned to fear them, and the sugar in them, when the foods that caused this confusion weren't even legitimate carbohydrates. They were fats in carbohydrate costumes.

You do not get fat from eating natural carbohydrates, even with sugar in them. You get fat from eating processed imitators with refined sugar added. Before we had processing — freezing, drying, canning, pickling, sweetening, preserving, coloring, texturizing — sugar wasn't a problem in our diets. Today, 70% of our foods are processed, and these foods have created a sugar excess in our diets. They've also dramatically increased our fat problems, because the combination of ingredients in refined foods is the formula that makes fat store easily.

This doesn't mean that all processed foods are bad for you. There are many new versions arriving in the supermarket every day. But don't be fooled by the names or claims. For instance, a cereal called *Natural Grain* might make you think it's made from whole grains and isn't fattening, but you can get 6 teaspoons of sugar in every cup, and no real fiber. You can see a food that claims: *Lower Sugar* on the box or can, but you have to ask, lower than what? Lower than it was when it jumped off the scale for sugar content, meaning it can still be too sugary and too fatty. And the term *natural* can be misleading when it refers to sugar, because double barrelled table sugar (sucrose) is allowed to be called natural, since it once occurred in beets and sugar cane. Even the processed diet foods can be high in sugar, giving you empty calories.

It's up to you to do some serious investigating of processed and refined foods with a magnifying glass in the supermarket, if you have to. It will save you pounds of fat and sugar each year.

Your best plan for dieting is to avoid them as much as possible since they can't give you the kind of fat burn that you get from fresh food. You can save fast-lane foods for emergency situations if you must, but only use fat-free, low sugar and low-sodium varieties. And even then, you're losing fiber.

Diet/Sugar Smarts

- Sugar in processed foods provides empty calories, meaning you get calories but no nutritional benefits. When you're on a limited calorie plan (say 1200 calories) and you eat 400 calories per day as sugar, you're sacrificing 400 calories you could eat in fat-burning, filling foods such as vegetables, pastas or grains. 400 calories in vegetables or grains is high nutrition. You get more for your calories and feel more satisfied too.

- Sugar-rich foods are usually fat-rich foods and non-fibrous foods. That combination adds up to weight gain, not weight loss.
- Sugar-rich foods usually include additives too. When you're on a diet, additives can cause symptoms that might not occur when you're eating more calories. It's best to avoid as many additives as you can.
- Because high-sugar foods have low or no fiber, they can be eaten in a flash, no chewing and minimal salivation. And no time for hunger to abate naturally from eating (it takes 20 minutes). You might get a quick sugar boost that causes your blood glucose to rise, then drop again quickly. This doesn't give you steady, dependable energy, and it doesn't keep hunger at bay for long.
- Food tolerance tests suggest that eating high-sugar diets dulls your sensitivity to fats. In other words, you can eat more fat without being aware of it. Part of this is related to taste and part habit, since fat and sugar often get double billing in low-nutrition foods. To stay on the lean side, make sugar one of the first habits you break.
- Don't cut sugar by increasing your use of artificial sweeteners. Long-term studies on aspartame aren't completed yet.

DON'T FORGET
THAT EATING TOO MUCH
SUGAR CAN GIVE YOU
THE EPINEPHRINE EFFECT
***See* Epinephrine.**

HOW SWEET IT IS

Current Average Use
1 cup per day
or 48 Teaspoons

PRIMARY SOURCES OF REFINED SUGARS

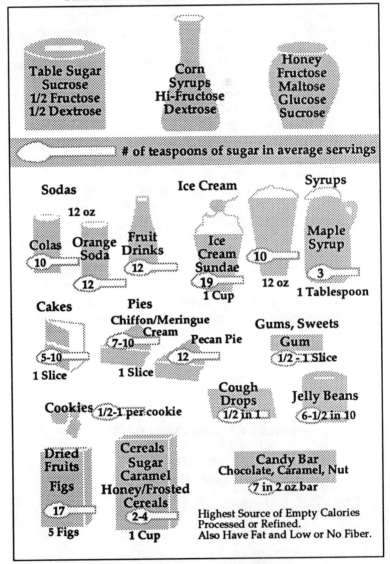

Empty Calories = 100% Sugar

RECOMMENDED DIET DOSE:
CUT INTAKE OF REFINED SUGAR
RELY ON FRESH FOOD SOURCES FROM FOOD GROUPS
SELECT OTHERS SPARINGLY

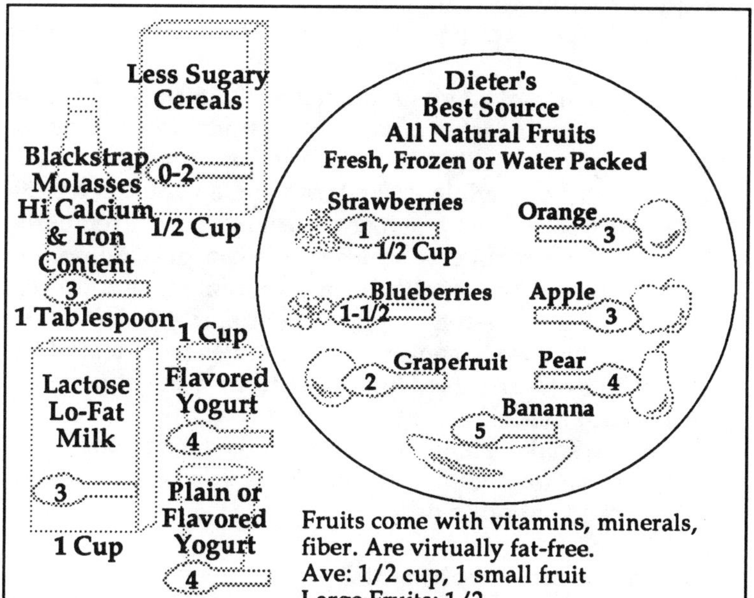

Fruits come with vitamins, minerals, fiber. Are virtually fat-free.
Ave: 1/2 cup, 1 small fruit
Large Fruits: 1/2

EZ LABEL GUIDE

Ingredients are listed on labels by weight. If sugar is first, the product is primarily sugar. If 2 or 3 sugars are midway on the list the product can be high sugar. If sugar is listed near the bottom, it's best.

Sugar	Invert Sugar
Sorbitol	Lactose
Sucrose	Malitol
Caramel	Maltose
Corn Syrup	Mannitol
Corn Syrup Solids	Molasses
Dextrose	Raw Sugar
Fructose	Turbinado
Honey	Xylitol

ARTIFICAL SWEETENERS*

ASPARTAME. 200 times sweeter than sugar. Synthetic. Combines 2 amino acids — aspartic acid and phenylalanine. Unstable in high heat such as baking. Not for people with Phenylketonia (metabolic disorder). Still being tested. Avoid or limit use to 1-2 servings daily.

»SACCHARINE 350 times sweeter than sugar. Synthetic. Studies link it to cancer.

* No indications that artificial sweeteners are beneficial to weight control.
» Not Safe

SUPPLEMENT, DIETS Powdered or Liquid Food Plans. Many diets are built around food supplements that act as meal replacements. These supplements can be liquid drinks in cans that are pre-mixed, powdered formulas in cans or packets that must be added to another liquid.

Advocates of food supplements claim they're a good way to get the benefits of a full meal (nutritionally), while avoiding the calories. A standard lunch might be 400 calories or more, while a standard supplement lunch is 50-100 calories. For fast lane people who don't eat regularly, and *won't* eat regularly, supplements can provide needed nutrition, but the quality of a supplement is a critical issue. If you are getting a lot of sugar along with reduced calories, the supplement isn't a good diet bet. Most of the supplements are used to provide low-fat sources of protein, but check the labels. If you're getting 5 grams of fat in one shake, along with sugar, this doesn't add up to dietary sense. Check the labels for additives or imbalanced amino acids.

Drawbacks To Supplement Diets

The problem with supplements for *dieters* are varied. They haven't got the metabolic clout of real food. Fiber content, if any, is minimal, and too many rely on sweeteners to make the food palatable. The right combination of amino acids is tricky and not sufficiently researched, and imbalances can occur. This can prevent the absorption of your protein, defeating the purpose of the supplement. In addition, you can start to rely on these supplements as food substitutes, which doesn't help you handle your real food issues. People develop emotional dependencies on supplements, seeing them as a form of medication, thinking they're responsible for the weight loss, which isn't true. It's the calorie restriction that is creating the weight loss, not the formula in the supplement. Most of the diets that use supplements are very low calorie ones, and that can promote rapid weight loss and rapid weight regain.

▲ **SWEET TOOTH** *Desire* for sweets, as opposed to a *need* for sweets. A part of emotional hunger. The more sweets you eat, the easier it is to tolerate higher levels of sugar. And the surprising fact is, that sweet tooth may be caused by a fat tooth in the background. Since sweet foods provide no real nutrition, you're wasting calories that you could get from fat burning foods such as complex carbohydrates. If you feel you must have sweets, make sure you're not using them in place of nutritious foods. First, insure that you're getting your daily food requirements met, then see if you have the room or desire for the sugary foods. You'll find that your desire for sugar will be decreased when you eat more fruits, vegetables, grains, and water. Balanced nutrition keeps that sweet tooth satisfied, not sweets. *See* Sugar. Fat Tooth.

SWEETENERS Sugars-natural and synthetic.*See* Sugar.

● **SWEETS** Sugar-rich foods such as candy, cola, ice cream, baked goods, processed foods. They provide empty calories and little nutrition, and are usually the foods you use to appease emotional hunger. Real hunger isn't abated by high-sugar foods. You get a quick rise in blood sugar, and a quick drop, and hunger returns quickly. Ten extra pounds per year can be attributed to high-sugar foods. The first step to slimness is to find substitutes for sugary foods that satisfy your desire for something sweet, while providing needed nutrition. Best substitute: fruit — something sweet and fat free with fiber, essential vitamins and minerals.

THE ESSENTIAL BIG MAC

◆ **SWIMMING** Aerobic exercise, non-weight bearing.
Benefits:
- Excellent cardiovascular training.
- Good calorie-burning exercise.
- No injury to joints.
- Works upper and lower body.
- Improves range of arm motion.
- Pools available at most community centers.
- Good exercise to combine with other activities.

t

◆ **TARGET HEART RATE** The recommended heartbeats/per minute that give you maximum oxygen uptake during aerobic exercise. This is considered cardiovascular conditioning, because it lowers your daily resting heart rate, which helps to avoid heart disease. The benefits are also muscular, since greater oxygen to your muscles increases their efficiency and increases your fat burn. Also called training rate.

The target heart rate zone is the range that is recommended for aerobic conditioning. It is 70-80% of your maximum heart rate. Figures for maximum heart rate were derived from stress tests on thousands of individuals, and the formula for target heart rate derived from those studies. Your maximum rate is not a *desired* rate, and if you find yourself nearing maximum, it's best to slow your heart beat by walking around the room, allowing it to decrease gradually. Sitting down or falling into an exhausted heap on the floor immediately after an aerobic exercise is not a safe way to bring your heart rate back to normal. A program of cool downs is usually the best routine to insure gradual heart rate recovery.

How To Measure Your Heart Rate.

Find your pulse on your wrist or neck, just below your jaw. Place your four fingers (not thumb) lightly over your pulse and count the number of beats for 10 seconds. Multiply that number by 6 (for 60 second rate).

Use your 60 second rate to compare to the table for target heart rate.

AGE	TARGET ZONE 70%	85% of Max	MAXIMUM HEART RATE Heart beats/min
20 (or under)	140	170	200
25	137	166	195
30	133	162	190
35	130	157	185
40	126	153	180
45	123	149	175
50	119	145	170
55	116	140	165
60	112	136	160
65 (or older)	90	132	155

HEART BEAT TOO FAST? You started too fast and are pushing too hard. Walk around the room to slow your heart beat. Don't sit to do it. You want to bring your heart beat down gradually. When you return to your exercise, keep it more fluid and steady. Don't strain or push yourself. *See* Interval Training.

◆ **TENNIS** Skill sport aerobic exercise (if you stay active). *See* Exercise.

● **THERMOGENESIS** The thermic effect of food, or heat from eating. Eating, digesting and absorbing food takes metabolic energy. You burn calories by eating too. Some foods cause a great rise in your metabolism, needing more energy to be broken down into the form for absorption by your blood. By choosing more thermic foods, you can burn 10-15% more calories each day.

Complex carbohydrates are very thermic foods. They use approximately 23 calories out of every 100 calories to be digested and absorbed. If you eat 700 calories of complex carbohydrates daily, you burn 161 calories because you ate them. To a dieter trying to lose fat, that's a significant amount of calories. Fat is barely thermic. It only uses 3 calories out of every 100 to digest and absorb. If you eat 400 calories of fat daily, that's only 12 calories burned from eating fat. The remaining 388 fat calories are easily stored. Protein is also a very thermic food, but it has a higher fat content than carbohydrates, and the fat can be stored. The leaner proteins are the best thermic bet.

▲ **THIN FROM WITHIN** Using your inner resources to help you achieve your weight loss goals. *See* Imagery.

TRACE MINERALS Organic or inorganic materials found in small amounts in your body, and also found in food. Some are essential. *See* Minerals.

◆ **TRAMPOLINE** Aerobic exercise device for rebounding. You can use a regular trampoline or a mini-trampoline for at-home rebounding.

Benefits:

- Excellent cardiovascular fitness.
- Great calorie-burning potential.
- Easily accommodates all levels of fitness.
- Develops coordination and balance.
- No injury to muscles and joints.

◆ **TREADMILL** Stationary aerobic exercise machine.

Benefits:

- Superb cardiovascular training.
- Excellent calorie-burning exercise.
- Great for all levels of fitness, accommodating beginners to seasoned exercisers.
- Available in motorized and manual (motorized is usually better for the beginner because there's less tension and the speed and grade are easy to adjust; manual machines are more appealing to the advanced

treadmiller because of the greater challenge of motorizing it yourself).

- Reduces body injury.

TRIGLYCERIDE Another name for lipid, or fat in your cells or blood.

TRYPTOPHAN An essential amino acid that occurs naturally in food proteins, such as meat, poultry, fish, peanuts and dairy. The naturally-occurring form of tryptophan is not only safe, but essential. It is one of the 8 amino acids that cannot be produced by your body and must be derived from your food.

● **TV DINNERS** Pre-portioned meals in heat-and-serve packages. These aren't the best foods to eat in front of the TV or anywhere else. They're usually low in fiber and high in sugar and fat. The TV is one of the major cues to eat, and an entire industry of microwave and oven entrees capitalized on that. Food commercials appear on TV every 15 minutes on most stations, and the models eating fats and sugars are always thin and toned. Most dieters are told to stop eating in front of the TV, and in a clinical world, that would be ideal. But home isn't a clinical world, and TV is a part of many people's lives. If you don't feel you can stop eating in front of the TV, adjust your couch eating to a healthy habit. Instead of eating a processed dinner, make your own variety of TV entrees and freeze them in one meal servings for reheating. You can make casseroles, pasta salads, stews, and soups with complex carbohydrate vegetables and grains. That way you won't have the extra fat, sugar and salt. This kind of TV dinner can make a couch potato lean.

U

▲ **UNDEREATING** Eating less than the required nutrition for healthy body maintenance. This can be a mild form of undereating for a few days, or a week of starvation. Either way, your body is malnourished, and over time, this leads to serious illnesses and metabolic disturbances. Undereating or starving for a few days is often perceived by dieters as a way to make up for days of eating poorly, or overeating. Dieters think that *not eating* will lead to faster weight loss. In fact, the reverse is true. Not eating, or nutrient starvation, will throw your body into a calorie-conserving state, and your metabolism will reduce in order to hold on to the few calories you eat. This causes you to burn less calories overall, and it forces your body to go after its own muscle protein for energy. Calcium is taken from your bones, muscle is broken down for protein, and you wind up with an undermined metabolism, and risk osteoporosis. You are less resistant to stress, which further depletes nutrient stores, and illness often results.

When undereating is prolonged, you will see weight loss, but it's water and muscle being wasted, and the appearance of this form of weight loss is dragged out, both externally and internally. In a literal sense, your body drags out every nutrient it can find before it goes after fat. You can remain fat and be depleted, which will lead to more fat gain. If more dieters understood this simple catch 22 about *not eating,* it would save them serious consequences in weight regain. In the end, undereating will lead to more fat gain.

UNDERWATER WEIGHING A method for determining body fat content, usually in major athletic centers. The method uses a tub of water that is attached to a scale. You get in the tub, and water is displaced. The more fat you have, the more water displacement, since fat is lighter than water. This makes the scale lighter and it lifts. Slimmer bodies sink lower because muscle is heavier than water. Your "water" weight is then compared to your dry weight to calculate your body fat content.

UNDERWEIGHT 10% below ideal body weight. Any weight loss beyond that degree is usually accompanied by physiological problems, particularly in women. Being underweight without lack of daily nutrients is generally considered safe, if not good prevention, since weight tends to increase with age. However, underweight with malnutrition is a serious condition making the person more susceptible to infections and disease. Underweight people who are malnourished lose muscle tissue, and a main priority should be replacing these losses. The recommended therapy is a well-balanced diet with extra protein to rebuild muscle tissue, frequent small meals, and exercise to gain muscle, not fat. The diet should not seek to increase the fat level, promoting fat gain as weight gain since the low muscle body will gain fat easily. An increase up to 500 calories per day is recommended in lean proteins, complex carbohydrates and low-fat dairy. The goal is to gain weight slowly, up to 1 pound per week. This is achieved by eating 500 more calories per day.

❤ **UNSATURATED FAT** The fat in food that is considered OK fat, since it helps reduce the level of LDL or bad cholesterol in your body. *See* Cholesterol.

V

● **VARIETY** Diversity in food energy, specifically from the four major food groups. When dietary guidelines suggest that you "eat a variety of foods," it has a very literal meaning. Not just any variety, but the *science of variety* furnished in the food group system, where foods are grouped according to their highest-yield nutrients. No two foods yield the same nutrients and many nutrients need to be in the presence of, or in combination with other nutrients to work properly. The science of variety insures that you receive 50 essential nutrients you need on a daily basis when you eat the required servings in each group – 2 servings Meat, 2 servings Milk, 4 servings Fruits & Vegetables, 4 servings Grain. This applies even if you are on a diet for weight loss. If you omit one or two groups during a diet, you could lose 1/4 to 1/2 of the nutrition your body needs on a daily basis to supply healthy, non-saggy fat loss.

Many dieters have the mis-impression that eating balanced meals is a tired idea, and they look instead to some magic food or magic combination of foods as the solution to their weight problems. The fact is, that may be a good reason why their weight problems continue. Eating for variety means eating for power and health.

The Benefits of Variety

- you get the protein you need for lean muscle protection – and that means better fat burn
- you get the fiber you need for fullness and better intestinal transit time – and that means less calorie absorption
- you get the 50 essential nutrients automatically – and that means health and disease prevention
- you get the calcium you need to prevent bone deterioration as you age
- you get the textures you need for chewing – and that means better appetite control
- you get pleasure from variety – it's more palatable, and less likely to make you break your diet from boredom
- you get an automatic maintenance plan – all you have to do is increase your calories across the board
- you're set for a healthy, slimmer life.

The science of variety is the real magic combination. *See* Food Groups.

● **VEGETABLES** Carbohydrate sources of fiber, vitamins and minerals. One of the food groups for healthy eating. Diet foods. *See* Food Groups.

▲ **VISUALIZATION** The ability to picture success before it occurs, in order to increase the likelihood that it will occur. *See* Imagery. Relaxation.

VITAMINS Organic nutrients from food that have no calories or energy. Vitamins are the building blocks of your enzymes — the chemicals needed to break down your foods for energy. Your body can't make most vitamins on its own, and they must be provided daily in your food. One of the reasons you eat for variety, and need all food groups to do it, is because no one food or group provides all of the essential vitamins in the ratios your body needs.

Your vitamin needs are based on many factors: your age, sex, health status, weight, genetics, stress level, activity level, and even the climate. For this reason, it's best to take the easy route and get them from your daily food, as recommended in the food groups. Trying to study vitamins and figure out isolated needs, could take a lifetime, and it often leads to confusion, if not vitamin excess.

There are two forms of vitamins—water soluble (can be excreted) or fat-soluble (can be stored). It's fairly easy to tell the difference. Fat-soluble vitamins like A,D, E, & K are measured in IUs (International Units)and that's listed on the label. Water soluble vitamins are measured in milligrams (mg) on labels.

More than 50 vitamins and nutrients are needed in the presence of water for healthy body balance. To make it easier to get them, 10 leader nutrients were identified as essential in your diet. When you get these leader nutrients, you automatically get the rest of your vitamins.

The ten leader nutrients were used to design the food groups. They are: Calcium, Carbohydrates, Protein, Fat, Vitamin A, C, B1 (Thiamin) and B2 (Riboflavin), Niacin and Iron.

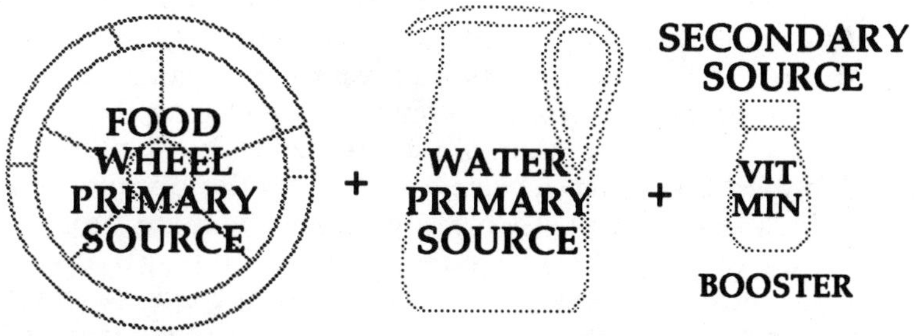

THE EASIEST WAY TO GET YOUR LEADER NUTRIENTS AND VITAMINS DAILY PLUS ALL MINERALS

The Vitamins

Vitamin A
Vitamin B Complex
- B1 Thiamine
- B2 Riboflavin
- B6 Pyridoxine
- B12
- B13 Orotic Acid
- Biotin
- Choline
- Folic Acid
- Inositol
- B17 Laetrile
- Niacin
- Para-Aminobenzoic (PABA)
- B15 Pangamic Acid
- Pantothenic Acid

Vitamin C
Vitamin D (Food and Sunlight)
Vitamin E Tocopherol
Vitamin F Unsaturated Fatty Acids
- Linoleic Acid
- Linoleic Acid
- Arachidonic Acid

Vitamin K
- Kl
- K2

Vitamin P
Biof lavonoids

VLCD Very low calorie diet. 600 calories (or less) per day. Also called hypocaloric diets. The most common variety of these diets are fasts, modified fasts, meal replacement diets, ketone diets, and often one-or-two food diets that dramatically limit your calories. The only way to make an 800 calorie (or less) diet meet the requirements for essential daily nutrients is to provide part or most of the diet in the form of a food substitute or meal replacement, which concentrates protein in a low-fat liquid or powder. These are rapid weight loss diets, and produce the effects associated with rapid weight loss — refeeding problems and rapid weight regain. Some studies indicate that they also produce greater hunger afterward, and can lead to bouts of binge eating that may not have been a problem in the pre-diet state. The one-or-two food diets that achieve a very low calorie format are imbalanced diet plans, often without adequate protein, which causes extreme muscle losses, and nutritional deficiencies. All very low calorie diets allow muscle losses to occur, and the weight regain that follows appears rounder as a result.

◆ **VOLLEYBALL** Skill sport aerobic exercise (if you keep moving). *See* Exercise.

W

◆ **WALKING** Low-impact aerobic exercise.

Walking develops muscle tone, strength, endurance, flexibility, and agility. Joggers say that running puts them in touch with their bodies, but walking goes one step further — it gives you time and space to reflect on yourself and your environment. The visual stimulation of walking is less stressful than jogging, with fast-forward films running across your eyes. You can enjoy nature or your city, noticing things that might otherwise have passed you by.

➡ **How To Do Aerobic Walking**

- In the beginning, duration is more important than distance.
- Begin with modest distances and gradually increase your speed as walking becomes more comfortable.
- Swing your arms rhythmically and try to breathe deeply.
- Strike the longest stride that is comfortable for you.
- Keep your momentum steady and think about being light, putting less weight on your feet.
- Wear light, comfortable clothes and shoes that don't slip or rub.

◆ **WARM UPS** A mild exercise or stretching routine for 8-10 minutes to precede strenuous exercise. If you've ever reached to one side too quickly and pulled a muscle, you know the effect that sudden movement can have on tight muscles – strain. This can happen when you jump into a vigorous workout routine or aerobic exercise without warming up. Tight muscles feel cold and your goal is to elongate them, which raises your body temperature, stimulates your circulation, giving you a warm feeling. This increases the efficiency of muscle contractions, and makes you more supple, protecting you from injury or strain. The increase in blood circulation is especially important to older or sedentary exercisers, because it prevents myocardial ischemia (insufficient blood supply to the heart). In a pinch, walking is an ideal warm up, or you can use an overall body stretch, flexing and relaxing one muscle group at a time, from your head to toe, while breathing deeply. Or you can follow the example of many athletes who prefer Yoga for a great overall stretch. *See* Cool Downs. Stretches. Yoga.

● **WATER** Essential body fluid. Also any liquid excreted from your body such as urine, sweat, tears.

Your body is about 60% water. Men tend to have 10% more body water than women. Slender man – 65% water; slender woman – 55% water. Obese people tend to have less body water than normal. Obese man – 55%; obese woman – 45%. 2/3 of your body water is located inside your cells, and the other 1/3 is outside your cells.

Your body water content is regulated by three mechanisms:

1. Thirst, which causes you to drink when your water level is low.
2. Pituitary Gland, which releases or withholds an anti-diuretic hormone (ADH) that acts as a water monitor and stabilizer.
3. Kidneys, which expel water and waste products.

You lose about 1/2 gallon of water each day, through sweating, body excretion and breathing. You can lose more than 1/2 gallon if you exercise, if outside temperature rises, or if you experience fever, vomiting or diarrhea.

YOUR GOAL:
TO REPLACE THE WATER YOU LOSE DAILY

The easiest way to insure that you get your daily water requirements is to fill 2 1-quart pitchers with water and make sure you drink them each day. Preferred – at least 2 glasses with each meal, and 2 in-between meals.

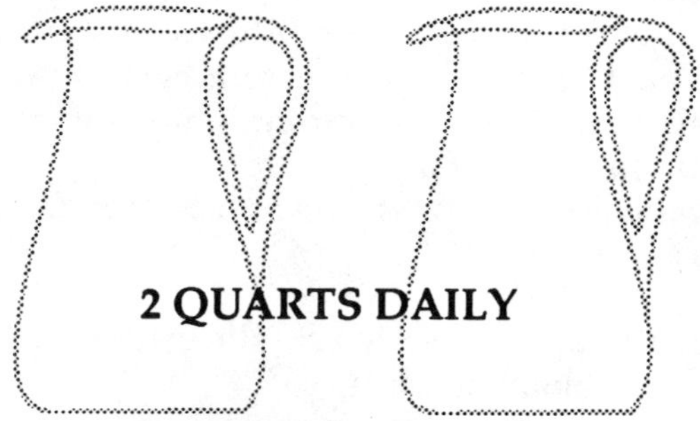

FOR FLUID BALANCE & FAT METABOLISM

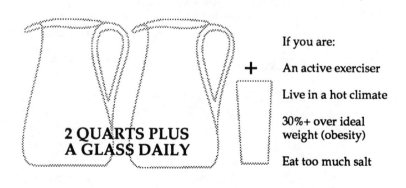

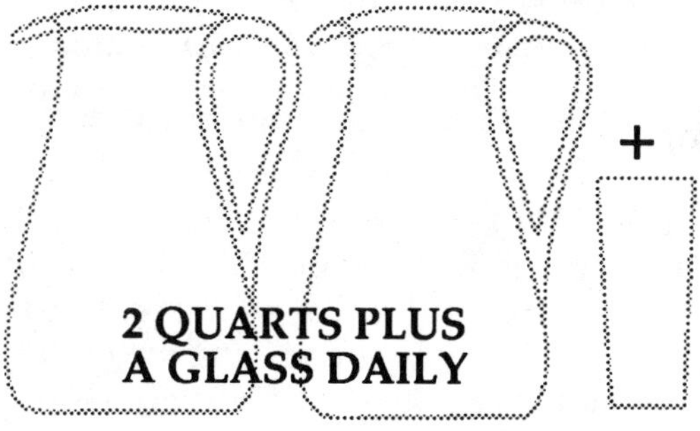

If you are:

An active exerciser

Live in a hot climate

30%+ over ideal weight (obesity)

Eat too much salt

THE MAGIC FORMULA – H_2O AND WHY YOU NEED IT FOR WEIGHT LOSS

- It improves your fat metabolism. More water leads to less fat stored.
- It suppresses your appetite. You can use it as a no- calorie snack.
- It's necessary for proper digestion.
- It binds with fiber to create a feeling of fullness.
- It acts as a natural diuretic to prevent water retention.
- It supplies oxygen to your muscles, which are the home of your fat burn. More oxygen means better metabolic fire. More water to your muscles means better muscle function, since muscles are 72% water.
- It maintains normal bowel function. This allows food to move through your intestines with ease, and prevents excess calories from being absorbed. The longer food stays in your intestines, the more calories you can store as fat.
- It removes wastes which are increased during weight loss.

❤ Water is vital to your heart, since it maintains blood volume and blood pressure.
NOTE: If you only drink water when you are thirsty, you are already in 2% dehydration. In a 130-lb. person, that means you are down 1-1/2 pounds of essential water. Don't wait until you are thirsty.

Drinking less water will not prevent water retention. In fact, the opposite is true. If you don't have enough body water, the hormone ADH will be released to act as a water-conservator.

WATER RETENTION Holding water. This is usually caused by excessive sodium intake or inadequate intake of drinking water, or both simultaneously. (Presuming absence of disease.) Diuretics are not advised for mild or periodic water retention in healthy people, since cutting back on salt and drinking more water is the best medicine.

Do not confuse mild water retention with Edema, which usually indicates an underlying disorder that needs specific medical attention. *See* Water. Sodium.

WEIGHT A combination of water, fat and muscle (lean body mass). Your basic body composition breaks down this way:

- Water is typically 55-60% of your total body weight.
- Fat ranges from 10-30+% of total body weight in women. Fat content can be lower, but it is rare and dangerous. Fat ranges from 8-25+% of total body weight in men (they have less fat to begin with).
- Muscle (stripped down muscle tissue and bone is the rest).

Muscle weight is also called LEAN BODY MASS and is usually measured along with water, muscle and bone, because they are difficult to separate. Muscles are approximately 72% water, while fat has very little water content — approximately 3%. Measurements of muscle, therefore, take in everything that is *not* fat, and is called your fat-free mass.

The ideal weight combination is low fat, high muscle and balanced water.

◆ **WEIGHT LIFTING** An exercise for muscle building or body building. The only caution, besides possible strain or injury, is to watch protein and fat levels. Excess fat in your diet can be a detriment to your results. Muscles can be built up under a layer of fat and the look appears too bulky. It also can inhibit your flexibility. It's best to combine muscle building with stretching exercises and a low fat diet, so the look is lean, toned muscular, and flexible.

WEIGHT LOSS Water, muscle or fat reduction. This is an important definition to keep in mind. Weight loss can be any of the three losses, but the only one you need is *fat loss.* Water facilitates fat removal, so losing water won't help you get slim. And water losses aren't *real* indicators of successful weight loss, since water displacement in early phases of a diet will eventually stabilize.

Muscle wasting is what you want to avoid on a diet, because muscle is the home for your fat to burn. The more muscle you lose, the greater your tendency to store and gain fat. This becomes very apparent in maintenance after a muscle-wasting diet, because you'll see your weight come back *fast*, and you'll be gaining only fat. Muscle wasting diets cause rapid weight regain that's hard to stop. One of the reasons men are good calorie burners is due to their higher content of body muscle. Women start out with a higher body fat content, and when muscle losses occur with dieting, they exacerbate fat problems.

The most common diets that can cause muscle losses are:

- imbalanced diets that rely on one or two foods as primary fuel, or diets with entire food groups missing
- starvation diets
- very low calorie diets
- diets with inadequate protein
- any combination of the above, without exercise

The two known ways to protect muscle during a diet are: (1) eating adequate food protein (along with a balanced diet). This prevents your body from going after your muscle protein to burn for energy. (2) Exercise. This protects existing muscle and builds new muscle for ideal weight maintenance. That's why the best diets advocate exercise at the start of calorie reduction.

WEIGHT MAINTENANCE Energy balance. Your output equals your input. You burn what you eat. *See* Maintenance for guidelines.

WEIGHT-RELATED Created by or associated with excess weight. This covers a wide spectrum of science, including diseases or disorders that are advanced by fat gain, personality issues that emerge from fat gain, habits and behavior that center around weight, in addition to any discipline that advances treatment. Specifically, this means factors that have been validated by research or clinical study to have a direct relationship with weight gain and weight loss. *See* Risks.

▲ **WELLNESS** Absence of disease. This means more than not having an illness. It means being in a health state that minimizes the risks of future illnesses which are lifestyle diseases — hypertension, diabetes, heart disease and cancer. The concept of wellness didn't quite catch on as a movement in health, and has been primarily used in the corporate sphere. It involves two phases: the evaluation phase and resolution phase.

The primary issues involved in a wellness evaluation are:

1. Weight Problems. Are you 10% away from your ideal body weight?
2. Energy Level. Are you tired, and do you lack stamina? Do you exercise regularly?
3. Habit Problems. Do you use medications or alcohol too frequently?
4. Stress Problems. Do you have difficulty concentrating, feel anxious, or have a quick temper. Are your sleep patterns regular?
5. Food Problems. Do you have digestion problems? Do you use diet aids or digestive aids frequently.

▲ **WILLPOWER** Mind over matter. The ability to use strength of mind to support your desires, wishes and goals. Too often, in dieters, this strength of mind is seen as the power to say NO. But that's not the whole story with willpower. It's also the ability to say YES. And it implies the ability to make self-enriching choices. The concept of willpower has been so abused with deprivation diets, that it isn't its old self. To get back to a state of self-initiation — the ability to drive yourself forward—use SKILLPOWER. This will help you regain your perspective on will, and simultaneously, it will drive you to your goal. One of the best skills a dieter can use is Relaxation Exercise, and its adjunct, how to turn negative thinking into positive thinking. To learn how to let go of the No's and substitute the YES's, see Rationalizations.

X Y Z

X FACTOR DIETS Programs that promote one vitamin, mineral, enzyme, amino acid, or an odd combination of them, as the cause for weight loss. Alphabet diets that use any letter to symbolize the unknown X. In mathematics, the x factor is a variable, a solution you can derive in a number of different ways, if you assign different numbers to the X. That holds true for X factor diets. These diets often use the words "secret formula" and "our laboratory," and they often rely on testimonials for promotion. These diets are no secret. The poorest ones only use an enzyme or vitamin in isolation, and the better ones are simply disguises for normal low fat diets. The danger is believing the claims about certain components taken in isolation, and used as a supposed cure-all. It fosters a fad mentality, which doesn't help you deal with weight problems from a realistic perspective. The worst ones cause serious problems from nutrient imbalance, the best ones make you think that something other than dieting is responsible for weight loss. It' a clever trick, but tricks are something dieters have had enough of. *See* Food Groups.

▲ **YO YO SYNDROME** Rapid weight loss followed by rapid weight regain, often to weights higher than the original weight. This syndrome is common to, if not created by very restrictive diets that last for several months. Why?

Drastic Calorie Reduction. When you go on a very low calorie diet for months or more, you are retraining your body to exist on fewer calories. Your body holds its energy in store, because it "reads" that it will not be receiving more. The pattern of your everyday eating gives your body its information for a "reading." When you suddenly increase your calories back to average levels (it doesn't have to be excessive levels), you see weight regain, because average levels are dramatic increases when compared to the calorie level your body has adjusted to eating and burning. Very low calorie diets can reduce your metabolic output by as much as 30%. That means you are teaching your body to get by on 600-800 calories per day. When you go off the diet, and eat 500 calories more per day (an average level of eating or dieting), you don't have any metabolic power to burn the new calories. They head for storage. You also have another problem that compounds the issue.

Lean Muscle Losses. Your body protein mass (lean body muscle) is reduced on very low calorie diets. You lose vital body muscle along with your fat. This creates imbalanced body composition, with a fat mass that is too high and muscle mass that is too low, even though you may be slimmer. With a low muscle body, you gain fat more rapidly. When you gain, you gain fat not muscle, and you could wind up with a very high fat body that has been trained to get by on 600-800 calories per day. Your weight gain gives you the appearance of being soft and round all over, because you have too much body fat and not enough body muscle. Your weight gain after a rapid weight loss diet *appears* plumper than average weight gain. Physiologically speaking, it is plumper. And there's another problem that compounds the issue.

Repeat Dieting. The second time around, your rate of weight loss is slower, because of your reduced metabolic rate. If you choose another very low calorie diet, you can escalate your problems and might not lose weight at all, even though you are only eating 600-800 calories. Your body reads less calories coming in, and it holds back its energy again.

How To Get Out Of The Yo Yo Cycle

If you are a person who has suffered with yo-yo cycling, your best course is to absolutely avoid drastic solutions, and bring your body back into shape in steps. This is called step goals, and it means losing ten pounds, then stabilizing, losing 10 more pounds and stabilizing, until you get down to your ideal weight. The diet you choose should be one with a higher calorie level, such as 1000-1200 calories, and it should be based on the following ratio of food energy:

Carbohydrates	Protein	Fat
60% of total calories	20% of total calories	20% of total calories

Be patient and persistent in your body re-training. You don't want to see rapid weight loss, because that led to your yo yo problems. You want to see slow, steady weight loss, which is fat loss, and you want to see a firmer appearance from your weight loss. The point to remember is that your body is very forgiving — when you give it the right energy and give it a way to output that energy — with exercise, it will reward you by functioning more normally. Top off your diet plan with strong behavior skills that will hold you in good stead for ideal weight maintenance. This will prevent you from falling back into old habits of mis-eating that helped to create your weight in the first place. *See* Food Groups.

◆ **YOGA** A specialized exercise which concentrates on slow, stretching movements performed in harmony with breathing. The discipline can range from beginner stretching to advanced techniques, all designed to relieve stress from the spine, elongate muscles, toning your entire body system. Yoga also increases the oxygen supply to your body and achieves the effects of relaxation. *See* Exercise.

ZERO FAT No fat calories. A dieter's dream food. Is a zero-fat food the perfect food? Not necessarily. Consider these zero fat foods; sugar, alcohol, coffee, tea. Foods can have no fat and be poor food choices because they provide no nutrients. Diet sodas have no fat, lots of sugar, and additives. They deplete your diet rather than enhance it. Perfect foods are the ones that provide the most nutrient density for the least calories. It's the quality of the total composition that counts. A food can have fat and still be an ideal source of nutrition, such as the proteins in meats. Fruits have sugar, but they're packed with vitamins and minerals, and are ideal sources of fiber, which helps to remove fat. Excess fat is a major problem in our diets, but it doesn't stand alone as the cause for body fat. *Not eating* complex carbohydrates and getting sufficient fiber is equally the cause of body fat, and is essential for lowering cholesterol, along with cutting fat. The point to remember is that no food, or source of energy, stands alone as the cause or cure of fat and fat-related disease. It's the balance of foods that solve fat problems, foods working in harmony to provide essential nutrients along with variety and pleasure, varied taste and texture. This provides the right ingredients to make a perfect diet for weight loss and a perfect diet for life.

Calorie Counter

These are estimated values of standard foods. Your average daily intake of protein and fat are important on a diet. Protein protects your muscle and fat needs to be limited, so you lose your stored fat.

Average Protein Daily 60-65 grams — Average Fat Maximum 30-35 grams

You should meet the protein *maximum* daily for muscle protection, and *not* exceed the fat maximum to get lean and healthy on a diet.

	AMT	PRO	FAT	CARB	CALS
Ale	8 0zs	T	0	8	100
Alexander	Cktl Gl	1	1	1	225
Alexander, Brandy	Cktl Gl	1	1	1	240
Allspice	1/8 Tsp	0	0	0	0
Almond Cake	1 Sm Serv	2	4	27	160
Almond Choc. Bar	1	1	10	17	150
Almond Coffee Cake	1 Serv	4	7	35	200
Almond Cookies	2 Med	T	2	9	50
Almond Extract	2 Tsps	0	0	0	6
Almond Fudge	1 In Sq	1	4	22	130
Almonds, Salted	12 Med	3	9	3	100
Anchovies	6	5	3	T	50
Anchovies, Canned	2 Ozs	11	6	T	100
Anchovy Paste	1 Tbsp	5	3	1	50
Angel Food Cake	1 Serv	3	T	22	110
Animal Crackers	6	1	1	12	50
Anise	1/8 Tsp	0	0	0	0
Anise Cookies	3 Sm	T	2	9	50
Anisette Cordial	1	0	0	7	80
Apple	1 Sm	T	T	11	75
Apple, Baked	1	T	T	47	200
Apple Betty	4 Ozs	2	4	34	175
Apple Butter	1 Tbsp	T	T	9	35
Apple Cake, Dutch	1 Serv	T	1	65	270
Apple Cobbler	1 Sm	1	2	44	200
Apple Crumb Cake	1 Serv	T	1	49	200
Apple Dumplings	1 Med	1	2	63	275
Apple Fritter	1	1	16	12	205
Apple Jelly	1 Tbsp	T	T	13	50
Apple Juice	4 Ozs	T	T	14	55
Apple on Stick	1	T	T	55	230
Apple Pie	1 Serv	3	11	42	275
Apple Pie a la Mode	1 Serv	4	19	58	425

	AMT	PRO	FAT	CARB	CALS
Apple Pie, Deep Dish	1 Serv	5	8	44	270
Apple & Raisin Salad	1/2 Cup	1	T	25	200
Apple Salad, Diced	1 Serv	T	T	18	80
Apple Sauce Bread	1 Sl	3	1	21	110
Apple Sauce Cake	1 Serv	4	12	63	400
Apple Sauce, Canned	4 Ozs	T	T	13	55
Apple Sauce, Fresh	4 Ozs	T	T	11	50
Apple, Stewed	1	T	T	29	120
Apple Strudel	1 Serv	3	9	34	225
Apple-Carrot Salad	4 Ozs	T	T	11	50
Applejack	1 Shot	T	T	0	100
Apricot	1	T	T	4	20
Apricot Brandy	Cord.	T	T	7	75
Apricot Cordial	1 Gl	0	0	7	75
Apricot Jam	1 Tbsp	T	T	14	50
Apricot Nectar	4 Ozs	T	T	17	65
Apricot Pie	1 Serv	3	11	31	250
Apricots, Candied	4 Ozs	T	T	96	380
Apricots, Canned w/syrup	4 Ozs	T	T	19	75
Apricots,Canned, Water	4 Ozs	T	T	10	40
Apricots, Dried	5 Sm. Hlvs.	1	T	13	60
Apricots, Frozen, Sweetened	4 Ozs	T	T	26	110
Arrowroot	1 Tbsp	T	T	8	30
Arrowroot Cookies	1	T	1	4	25
Arrowroot Flour	2 Ozs	8	1	40	200
Artichoke	1 Med	2	T	10	50
Asparagus	4 Ozs	3	T	3	20
Asparagus, Canned	4 Ozs	3	T	3	20
Asparagus, (Cream Soup)	4 Ozs	3	1	9	60
Asparagus, Frozen	4 Ozs	3	T	3	25
Aspic Seafood	1 Serv.	34	2	2	170
Aspic Tomato	1 Serv	T	T	9	35
Aspic Tomato Salad	4 Ozs	4	T	4	40
Avocado	4 Ozs	2	18	7	190
Bacon, Canadian, Broiled	2 Ozs	16	10	T	155
Bacon, Crisp	3 Strips	5	8	T	100
Bacon Fat	1 Tsp	2	4	1	50
Bacon, Lettuce & Tomato	1 Av	10	10	29	245
Bagel	1	2	1	23	110
Baked Alaska	1 Serv	8	14	26	350
Baked Beans	4 Ozs	8	T	24	135
Baking Powder	1 Tap	T	T	2	10
Bamboo Shoots	4 Ozs	3	T	5	30
Banana	1 Med	1	T	23	95
Banana Bread	1 Sl	4	2	22	120
Banana Cake	1 Serv	2	5	36	200
Banana Cream Pie	1 Serv	5	8	56	300

	AMT	PRO	FAT	CARB	CALS
Banana, Fried	1 Med	1	6	35	200
Banana Split	1 Av	8	25	75	560
Barbecue Sauce	1 Tbsp	2	5	T	50
Barley	4 Ozs	10	1	80	390
Basil	1/8 Tsp	0	0	0	0
Bay Leaf	1/4 Tsp	0	0	0	0
Bean Sprouts (Mung)	4 Ozs	4	T	7	40
Bean Sprouts (Soy)	4 Ozs	8	5	8	115
Beans Look up by name					
Beef, Boiled	2 Ozs	17	4	0	110
Beef, Chuck (Pot Roast)	2 Ozs	16	8	0	145
Beef, Corned	2 Ozs	20	5	0	125
Beef, Dried	2 Ozs	19	4	0	115
Beef, Filet Mignon	2 Ozs	18	4	0	125
Beef, Flank, Cooked	2 Ozs	17	4	0	110
Beef, Hamburger	2 Ozs	14	11	0	160
Beef Heart	2 Ozs	17	3	0	105
Beef Kidney	2 Ozs	18	7	1	142
Beef Liver, Broiled	2 Ozs	11	2	3	80
Beef, Porterhouse Steak	2 Ozs	17	5	0	122
Beef Pot Pie	2 Ozs	5	8	10	137
Beef, Rib Roast	2 Ozs	16	28	0	148
Beef, Round Steak	2 Ozs	11	6	0	100
Beef, Short Ribs, Braised	2 Ozs	11	6	0	100
Beef, Sirloin Tip	2 Ozs	18	6	0	124
Beef Steak	2 Ozs	11	6	0	100
Beef Steak, Flank	2 Ozs	11	6	0	100
Beef Stew	2 Ozs	3	2	3	50
Beef, T Bone Steak	2 Ozs	17	5	0	122
Beef, Tenderloin Steak	2 Ozs	17	6	0	120
Beef Tongue	2 Ozs	9	8	T	112
Beer	12 Ozs	T	0	13	125
Beet Greens	1 Cup	2	T	4	25
Beet Sugar	1 Tbsp	0	0	4	18
Beets	4 Ozs	2	T	10	50
Beets, Cooked	4 Ozs	1	T	8	35
Benedictine	1 Oz	0	0	7	75
Bisquick Flour	4 Ozs	8	16	74	480
Bitter Chocolate	1 Oz	3	14	8	170
Black Beans	1 Serv	25	2	68	380
Blackberries, Canned	1 Cup	1	T	13	60
Blackberries, Fresh	1 Cup	1	1	13	60
Blackberry Brandy	Shot	0	0	0	75
Blackberry Pie	1 Serv	3	12	38	275
Bleu Cheese Salad Dressing	1 Serv	T	7	1	70
Blintzes, Cheese	1 Av	20	6	8	175

	AMT	PRO	FAT	CARB	CALS
Blintzes, Jelly	1 Av	4	6	35	210
Bloody Mary	1 Serv	1	T	5	95
Blueberries, Fresh	1 Cup	T	T	17	60
Blueberries, Frozen, Sweetened	4 Ozs	1	T	37	120
Blueberries, Frozen, Unsweetened	4 Ozs	1	T	22	60
Bologna	2 Ozs	8	14	T	165
Bon Bons	1	T	T	9	35
Bouillon Clear Condensed	4 Ozs	4	T	0	30
Bouillon Cubes	1	T	T	0	2
Boysenberries, Canned	4 Ozs	T	T	10	40
Boysenberries, Frozen, Sweetened	4 Ozs	T	T	27	110
Boysenberries, Frozen, Unswtnd	4 Ozs	1	T	13	55
Bran	1 Cup	8	2	32	111
Bran Flakes (40% Bran)	1/2 Cup	5	1	39	145
Brandy	3 Ozs	0	0	0	225
Brandy Fruit Cake	Av Serv	3	9	64	350
Bread, White, See Type	1 Sl	2	T	12	65
Brewer's Yeast, Dry	1 Tbsp	5	T	3	50
Brioche, Fr.	1	5	10	13	150
Broccoli	4 Ozs	3	T	5	30
Broccoli, Frozen	4 Ozs	5	T	6	35
Broccoli Soup	1 Serv	3	T	5	25
Broth, Clam	4 Ozs	3	T	T	20
Brussels Sprouts	1 Cup	5	T	9	50
Butter	1 Tbsp	T	11	T	100
Butter Cake	1 Serv	3	8	10	200
Butter, Salt	1 Tbsp	T	11	T	100
Butter, Sweet	1 Tbsp	T	11	T	100
Butterscotch Candy	1	1	3	24	120
Butterscotch Cookies	1	3	8	15	140
Cabbage, Baked	1 Serv	1	T	5	20
Cabbage, Chinese	15	T	T	3	1
Cabbage, Cole Slaw	4 Ozs	1	9	7	110
Cabbage, Raw, Shredded	1 Cup	1	T	5	25
Cake, Angel Food	1 Sl	3	T	22	110
Cake, Flour	1 Cup	9	T	85	380
Cake, Gingerbread	Av Serv	2	6	21	180
Cake, Pound	1 Sl	3	6	35	380
Cantaloupe	1/2 Melon	1	T	8	35
Caper Sauce	1 Tbsp	T	2	T	20
Capon	2 Ozs	12	12	0	160
Caramel Candies	1 Med	1	3	8	60
Caramel Choc. Nut Candy	1 Av.	2	3	32	165
Caramel Ice Cream Sundae	4 Ozs	5	10	28	215
Caramel Pudding	4 Ozs	3	5	29	170
Carbonated Water, Quinine	4 Ozs	0	0	9	35

	AMT	PRO	FAT	CARB	CALS
Carbonated Water, Seltzer	4 Ozs	0	0	0	0
Carrot Juice	1 Cup	T	T	13	50
Carrot Soup	1 Serv	T	T	10	45
Carrots, Canned	1 Cup	1	1	10	45
Carrots, Cooked	1 Cup	1	T	10	45
Carrots, Frozen	1/2 Cup	T	T	5	25
Carrots, Raw, Grated	1/2 Cup	1	T	3	20
Carrots, Raw, Sticks	3	T	T	3	14
Catsup	1 Tbsp	T	T	4	15
Cauliflower	1 Cup	3	T	5	30
Cauliflower , Frozen	1 Cup	4	T	8	50
Cauliflower , Soup	1 Cup	5	T	8	50
Celery, Cooked	4 Ozs	1	T	3	15
Celery, Raw	4 Ozs	1	T	4	20
Cereal, Bran Buds	1 Cup	7	1	44	144
Cereal, Cheerios	1 Cup	3	1	18	99
Cereal, Cornflakes	1 Cup	2	T	21	95
Cereal, Cream of Wheat	1 Cup	5	1	40	180
Cereal, Dry (Average)	1 Cup	2	T	15	100
Cereal, Oatmeal (Cooked)	132	2	23		5
Cereal, Raisin Bran	1 Cup	5	T	33	160
Cereal, Shredded Wheat	1 Biscuit	3	1	23	105
Cereal, Wheat, Bite Size	2 Ozs	6	1	30	200
Cereal, Wheat Germ	2 Ozs	17	6	28	220
Cereal, Wheat Whole (Average)	4 Ozs	2	T	11	50
Cereal, Whole Bran	1 Cup	4	T	32	120
Cereals: Check labels, many variations.					
Champagne	1 Gl	1	5	11	80
Cheddar Cheese, Grated	1/2 Oz	4	5	T	60
Cheddar Cheese, Processed	1 Oz	7	9	T	105
Cheese, American	1 Oz	6	9	T	100
Cheese, Bleu	1 Oz	5	8	T	100
Cheese, Camembert	1 Oz	4	6	T	80
Cheese, Cheddar	1 Oz	8	10	T	120
Cheese, Cheddar, Grated	1/2 Oz	4	5	T	60
Cheese, Cottage, Skim	1 Oz	5	T	1	25
Cheese, Cream	1 Oz	1	3	T	35
Cheese, Dry Grated	1 Tbsp	5	3	T	50
Cheese, Edam	1 Oz	9	13	2	125
Cheese, Fondue	1 Serv	20	21	9	315
Cheese, Limburger	1 Oz	6	8	T	100
Cheese, Parmesan, Grated	1 Oz	10	7	T	105
Cheese Sauce	1/2 Cup	11	18	5	225
Cheese Souffle	1/2 Cup	11	19	6	240
Cheese Spread	1 Oz	6	8	2	100
Cheese Spread, Bacon	1 Oz	10	9	2	130

	AMT	PRO	FAT	CARB	CALS
Cheese Sticks	2 Ozs	6	16	3	240
Cheese, Swiss	1 Oz	8	8	T	105
Cheese, Swiss Gruyere	1 Oz	8	8	T	110
Cheese, Velveeta	1 Oz	6	9	T	105
Cheeseburger sandwich	1 Av	28	37	22	540
Cherries, Candied, Choc.	2 Ozs	T	T	43	180
Cherries, Canned	1 Cup	1	T	19	90
Cherries, Fresh Pitted	1 Cup	1	T	20	85
Cherries, Maraschino	2 Av	T	T	2	10
Cherry Pie	1 Pc	3	15	41	350
Cherry Soda	8 Ozs	0	0	28	110
Chestnuts, Dried	8 Med	1	1	11	50
Chestnuts, Fresh	4 Ozs	3	2	47	220
Chicken, Baked	2 Ozs	10	9	0	125
Chicken, Barbecued	2 Ozs	12	7	T	112
Chicken, Boiled	2 Ozs	11	7	0	112
Chicken, Canned, Boned	2 Ozs	17	5	0	114
Chicken, Creamed	1/2 Cup	32	26	6	385
Chicken Fat	1 Tbsp	0	5	0	45
Chicken Giblets	2 Ozs	9	1	T	55
Chicken Giblets, Fried	2 Ozs	70	6	2	135
Chicken Gizzard, Cooked	2 Ozs	15	2	0	77
Chicken Gravy	2 Tbsp	T	9	4	100
Chicken Gumbo	4 Ozs	1	T	3	25
Chicken Heart, Cooked	2 Ozs	13	4	T	97
Chicken Liver, Chopped	2 Ozs	6	28	4	290
Chicken Pot Pie	2 Ozs	3	6	10	170
Chicken, Roasted	2 Ozs	17	3	0	105
Chicken Soup and Matzoh Balls	1 Cup	1	5	34	175
Chicken Soup, Creamed	1 Cup	1	3	4	45
Chicken Soup, Noodle	1 Cup	3	2	6	55
Chicken Soup w/Rice	1 Cup	2	1	6	45
Chip Beef	2 Ozs	19	4	0	110
Chitterlings, Fried	1 Serv.	16	20	0	250
Chives	1 Oz	T	T	1	5
Choc. Bar	1 Oz	2	9	16	150
Choc. Bar w/Nuts	1 Oz	3	10	17	170
Choc. Bitter	1 Oz	3	14	8	170
Choc. Butter Frosting	1 Tbsp	3	4	6	70
Choc. Cake, Iced	1 Sl	5	8	45	275
Choc. Candies, Sweet	1 Oz	1	11	18	170
Choc. Chiffon Pie	1 Pc	5	11	33	250
Choc. Chip Cookies	3 Med	2	6	22	150
Choc. Cookies	3	2	6	22	150
Choc. Covered Almonds	1 Oz	3	10	14	160
Choc. Covered Ice Cream	Av. Scp.	6	14	23	245

	AMT	PRO	FAT	CARB	CALS
Choc. Cream Cookies	1 Oz	4	5	20	140
Choc. Cream Peppermint Candies	1 Oz	4	5	8	110
Choc. Cream Pie	1 Pc	10	15	47	360
Choc. Creams	1 Av	2	2	12	60
Choc. Cup Cakes	1	2	7	20	155
Choc. Filling	1 Serv.	5	12	25	240
Choc. Finger Cookies	1 Serv.	5	8	6	115
Choc. Frosting	1 Tbsp	T	3	6	50
Choc. Fudge	1 Oz	T	5	27	125
Choc. Kisses, Candies	1	2	2	2	20
Choc. Layer Cake	1 Pc	5	5	64	320
Choc. Marshmallow Cookies	1	2	3	9	65
Choc. Marshmallow Pudding	4 Ozs	5	13	37	280
Choc. Mint Sauce	1 Serv	1	2	53	230
Choc. Mints	8 Sm	2	5	21	140
Choc. Mints Cream	1 Bar	4	6	23	160
Choc. Pudding	1/2 Cup	5	12	31	250
Choc. Sauce	1 Tbsp	1	1	5	25
Choc. Semi-Sweet	1 Bar	6	12	17	200
Choc. Skim Milk	1 Cup	7	5	26	170
Choc. Soda	8 Ozs	0	0	15	75
Choc. Syrup	1 Tbsp	T	T	10	35
Choc. Unsweetened	1 Sq	3	15	8	180
Choc. Wafer Cookies	1	2	1	6	40
Chop Suey, Beef	1/2 Cup	20	20	4	275
Chop Suey, Chicken	1/2 Cup	12	8	4	135
Chop Suey, Pork	1/2 Cup	12	8	4	135
Chop Suey, Vegetable	1/2 Cup	12	15	4	200
Chow Mein, Beef	1/2 Cup	14	4	2	115
Chow Mein, Chicken	1/2 Cup	14	4	2	110
Chow Mein, Pork	1/2 Cup	14	4	2	110
Chutney	1 Tsp	1	T	6	25
Cider	1 Cup	T	T	25	100
Cider, Apple	4 Ozs	T	T	13	55
Cider, Apple Hard	Shot	T	T	19	100
Cider, Sweet Apple	1 Cup	T	T	25	110
Cinnamon	1/8 Tsp	0	0	0	0
Cinnamon Bread	1 Sl	5	T	16	90
Cinnamon Bun	1	3	3	19	115
Cinnamon Cake	1 Sl	3	3	28	150
Cinnamon Muffin	1	2	4	23	135
Cinnamon Raisin Buns	1	2	4	29	160
Cinnamon Roll	1	5	4	11	100
Cinnamon Stick	1	0	0	0	0
Cinnamon Toast	1 Sl	7	6	29	200
Clam Chowder, Manhattan	1/2 Cup	0	0	2	30

	AMT	PRO	FAT	CARB	CALS
Clam Chowder, New England	1 Cup	2	6	4	95
Clam Dip, Sour Cream	3 Tbsps	14	16	T	200
Clam Juice	4 Ozs	3	T	0	20
Clam & Tomato Broth	1 Serv.	1	1	8	40
Clam & Tomato Soup	4 Ozs	1	1	6	35
Clams, Broiled	6	10	6	5	115
Clams, Broiled Stuffed	1 Serv	10	8	8	145
Clams (Canned) Drained	4 Ozs	17	3	2	105
Clams, Cherry Stone (Meat Only)	6	15	2	5	100
Clams, Fried	6	12	15	5	200
Clams, Raw	4 Ozs	15	2	4	90
Clams, Roasted	6	15	6	5	135
Clams, Steamed	4 Ozs	12	3	4	100
Clams, Stuffed, Baked	6 Sm	5	5	10	100
Clams, Stuffed, Deviled	6	5	5	10	100
Cobblers, All	1	1	2	44	200
Cocoa, Powder	1 Tbsp	T	T	8	32
Cocoa, Skim Milk	1 Cup	7	T	12	100
Cocoa Syrup	1 Tbsp	T	T	12	40
Cocoa, Whole Milk	1 Cup	7	7	18	165
Coconut Cake	Av Serv	3	7	29	200
Coconut, Dried, Sweetened	2 Ozs	2	20	27	280
Coconut, Dried, Unsweetened	2 Ozs	4	35	13	385
Coconut, Fresh	2 Ozs	2	20	11	210
Coconut Fudge	1" Sq	2	3	22	120
Coconut Macaroons	2 Sm	3	5	14	100
Coffee, Black	1 Cup	T	T	T	2
Coffee Cake	1 Pc.	3	4	14	105
Coffee Cake Iced w/nuts	1 Pc	4	10	33	240
Coffee Cream	1 Tbsp	T	3	1	30
Coffee, Expresso	2 Ozs	0	0	0	0
Coffee, Instant	1 Cup	T	T	0	2
Coffee, Turkish	1 Cup	T	0	20	100
Coffee, Viennese	1 Cup	T	2	8	50
Coffee w.Sugar, 1 Tsp	1 Cup	T	T	4	20
Coffee w/1 Tbsp. Condensed Milk	1 Cup	3	3	16	100
Coffee w/1 Tbsp. Evaporated Milk	1 Cup	1	1	2	20
Coffee w/1 Tbsp. Milk	1 Cup	T	T	T	10
Coffee w/1 Tbsp. Skim Milk	1 Cup	T	T	T	7
Coffee w/Cream	1 Cup	T	3	1	30
Coffee w/Sugar & Cream	1 Cup	T	T	5	50
Cognac	1 Oz	0	0	0	75
Cola	8 Ozs	0	0	25	100
Collards	1/2 Cup	2	2	5	45
Condensed Milk Sweetened	4 Ozs	9	9	60	330
Consomme (Clear)	1 Cup	4	T	0	30

	AMT	PRO	FAT	CARB	CALS
Cookies, Plain	1 Med	T	3	7	55
Cooking Fats	1 Tbsp	0	12	0	110
Cooking Oils (Vegetable)	1 Tbsp	0	14	0	125
Cooler, Rum	8 Ozs	4	6	19	150
Cooler Vermouth	1 Serv.	2	2	15	85
Cooler, Wine	8 Ozs	8	8	11	150
Cordials	Av Gl	0	0	7	75
Coriander	1/2 Tsp	0	0	0	0
Corn	2 Ozs	4	1	24	95
Corn Bread	1 Slice	4	5	22	170
Corn (Canned)	1 Cup	5	1	41	190
Corn Cereal, Puffed	2 Ozs	4	2	50	240
Corn, Cream of Soup	1 Cup	5	15	18	225
Corn Flour, Dry Sifted	4 Ozs	9	3	85	405
Corn Fritters	4 ozs	9	24	43	425
Corn, Frozen	4 Ozs	4	1	23	115
Corn Meal	1/2 Cup	5	2	45	230
Corn, Mexican Style	1/2 Cup	1	2	16	85
Corn Oil	1 Tbsp	0	14	0	125
Corn on the Cob	1 Sm	3	1	20	100
Corn Pone	2" Sq	4	3	40	210
Corn Starch	1 Tbsp	1	1	9	50
Corn Syrup	1 Tbsp	T	T	12	50
Corned Beef	2 Ozs	20	5	0	125
Corned Beef Hash	2 Ozs	8	4	4	73
Cotton Seed Oil	1 Tbsp	T	14	0	125
Crab, Canned	2 Ozs	10	T	0	56
Crab, Deviled	2 Ozs	9	1	0	52
Crab Meat	2 Ozs	13	2	T	70
Crab, Shelled	2 Ozs	10	1	T	50
Crabapples	1 Lg	T	1	7	90
Cranberries	4 Ozs	T	T	11	50
Cranberry Juice Cocktail	4 Ozs	T	T	18	75
Cranberry Relish	1 Tbsp	T	T	15	65
Cranberry Sauce	1 Tbsp	T	T	9	35
Cream, Half & Half	1/2 Cup	4	13	5	160
Cream, Heavy	1/2 Cup	2	42	3	410
Cream, Heavy	1 Tbsp	T	5	T	50
Cream, Light	1/2 Cup	2	23	5	235
Cream, Light	1 Tbsp	T	3	T	30
Cream Pie	1 Pc	22	13	50	405
Cream Pie, Boston	1 Pc	6	11	55	325
Cream Pie, Cherry	1 Pc	20	20	55	480
Cream Puff	2 Ozs	4	7	12	130
Cream Sauce	2 Tbsp	3	4	2	50
Cream Soda	6 Ozs	0	0	21	75

	AMT	PRO	FAT	CARB	CALS
Cream, Sour	1 Tbsp	T	3	T	30
Cream, Whipped	2 Tbsps	1	12	1	115
Creamer, Non Dairy	1 Tsp	T	T	1	10
Creme de Cocoa	Shot	0	0	7	75
Creme de Menthe	Shot	0	0	7	75
Crepe Suzettes	1 Av	10	12	22	235
Crisco	1 Tbsp	0	14	0	125
Croutons	6 Av	2	2	3	35
Crullers	1 Med	3	10	19	180
Crumb Cake	1 Sl	2	4	20	125
Crumb Cake, Apple	1 Pc	T	1	49	200
Crumbs, Bread	1 Tbsp	6	2	4	60
Crust, Pie Graham Cracker	Bottom	4	19	64	450
Cucumber	8"	T	0	3	14
Cumin	1/8 Tsp	0	0	0	0
Cupcake	1 Med (2 ozs)	2	6	33	95
Currants, Dried	4 Ozs	5	2	74	160
Currants, Fresh	2 Ozs	1	T	5	30
Curry Powder	1 Tsp	0	0	0	0
Custard	1/2 Cup	3	3	24	130
Custard, Banana	1 Serv	6	6	24	175
Custard, Butterscotch	1 Serv	5	5	12	125
Custard (Canned) Instant	1 Serv	6	3	23	125
Custard, Egg, Baked	1/2 Cup	10	6	14	160
Custard, Frozen	4 Ozs	5	12	20	210
Custard Pie	1Sl	6	12	23	225
Custard Sauce	1 Tbsp	6	6	2	85
Custard, Vanilla, Frozen	4 Ozs	5	12	20	210
Daiquiri	Cktl Gl	0	0	7	75
Dandelion Greens	4 Ozs	3	T	9	55
Danish Pastry	2 Ozs	4	13	25	240
Date Cookies	2	4	3	15	110
Date & Nut Bread	1 Sl	2	1	21	100
Dates, Dried	1 Cup	4	1	13	560
Dates, Pitted	1/2 Cup	2	T	67	275
Dates, Pitted Candies	1 Bar	2	3	20	110
Devil's Food Cake	1 Sl	2	8	32	210
Deviled Egg	2	20	15	2	225
Deviled Ham	1 Tbsp	10	10	T	130
Deviled Ham Spread	1 Serv	5	10	T	110
Diet Dressings	1 Tbsp	T	2	1	25
Dill Pickles	1 Av	T	T	2	5
Dixie Cup	1 Cup	6	14	20	230
Dixie Cup Sundae	1 Serv	6	14	53	365
Doughnut, French	1 Oz	4	14	21	225
Doughnut, Iced	1 Oz	3	10	37	230

	AMT	PRO	FAT	CARB	CALS
Doughnut, Jelly	1 Oz	3	10	37	245
Doughnut, Plain	1 Oz	3	10	19	180
Doughnut, Sugared	1 Oz	3	10	21	185
Duck Eggs	1 Med	6	5	1	75
Duck, Roasted	2 Ozs	11	4	0	95
Dumplings	1 Med	1	2	19	100
Eclair, Choc. (Creamed)	1 Av	7	15	15	225
Eclair, Choc. (Custard)	1 Av	7	15	20	240
Eels, Raw	2 Ozs	9	10	0	130
Eels, Smoked	2 Ozs	10	15	0	183
Egg	1 Med	6	6	T	80
Egg, Poached	1 Av	6	6	1	80
Egg White	1	3	0	T	10
Egg Yolk	1	3	6	T	80
Eggplant	1 Sl	1	T	7	35
Eggs, Deviled	2	20	15	2	225
Eggs, Dried	1 Tbsp	3	3	T	40
Eggs, Duck	1 Med	6	5	1	75
Eggs, Florentine	1 Serv	14	14	4	200
Eggs, Fried	1 Med	6	8	T	95
Eggs, Scrambled	2	11	12	T	155
Endive	4 Ozs	1	T	4	25
English Toffee	1 Pc	T	T	13	56
Escarole	4 Ozs	1	T	4	25
Eskimo Pie	Av	3	6	32	205
Fennel	1/8 Tsp	0	0	0	0
Feta Cheese	1 Oz	6	8	T	100
Fig Bars	1 Lg	1	1	19	90
Fig Newton	2	1	1	22	100
Figs (Canned)	4 Ozs	T	T	19	75
Figs, Dried	1	1	T	12	55
Figs, Fresh	4 Sm	1	T	24	100
Filet Mignon	2 Ozs	18	4	0	125
Fish, Abalone	2 Ozs	10	T	1	50
Fish, Blue Baked	2 Ozs	12	5	0	115
Fish, Blue Fried	2 Ozs	11	2	0	112
Fish Cakes, Fried	2 Ozs	8	4	5	95
Fish Chowder	1 Cup	1	2	12	65
Fish, Cod	2 Ozs	9	T	0	40
Fish, Cod (Cakes)	2 Ozs	8	4	5	94
Fish, Flounder	2 Ozs	9	T	0	45
Fish, Gefuelte	1 Serv	3	2	1	75
Fish, Haddock	2 Ozs	10	3	4	90
Fish, Halibut	2 Ozs	10	3	0	70
Fish, Herring	1 Sm	26	8	0	190
Fish, Herring,Kippered	1 Sm	22	13	0	190

	AMT	PRO	FAT	CARB	CALS
Fish, Lobster	1/2 Avg	16	2	T	90
Fish, Lobster, Canned	2 Ozs	10	1	T	55
Fish, Mackerel, Canned	2 Ozs	10	6	0	95
Fish, Salmon	2 Ozs	9	9	0	125
Fish, Salmon, Canned	2 Ozs	10	7	0	110
Fish, Sardines, Canned	2 Ozs	15	6	0	115
Fish, Shad	2 Ozs	10	5	0	90
Fish, Shrimp, Canned	2 Ozs	15	1	0	70
Fish, Sole	2 Ozs	18	7	0	90
Fish, Swordfish	2 Ozs	15	4	0	100
Fish, Tuna, See Tuna	2 Ozs	15	4	0	102
Flour, All Purpose	1 Cup	12	1	84	400
Flour, Arrowroot	2 Ozs	8	1	40	200
Flour, Bisquick	4 Ozs	8	16	74	480
Flour, Buckwheat	1 Cup	6	1	80	350
Flour, Cake	1 Cup	9	T	85	380
Flour, Corn Meal	1 Cup	11	4	90	460
Flour, Rye, Dark	1 Cup	20	3	76	410
Flour, Rye, Light	1 Cup	11	1	98	440
Flour, Soy Bean (Full Fat)	1/2 Cup	41	23	41	505
Flour, Soy Bean (Low Fat)	1/2 Cup	49	7	34	425
Flour, Wheat	1 Cup	13	1	84	400
Flour, White	1 Cup	12	1	84	400
Fondue, Cheese	1 Serv	20	21	9	315
Frankfurter	1 Av	5	11	T	120
Frankfurter, All Beef	1 Av	7	14	0	170
Frankfurter Rolls	1 Av	7	6	12	160
Frankfurters & Sauerkraut	1 Serv	8	14	5	200
Frappe, Ice Cream	10 Ozs	12	19	35	360
French Fried Potatoes	6 Av	1	5	12	100
French Onion Soup	1/2 Cup	5	2	5	60
French Pastry	Med	4	9	40	260
French Rolls	1 Av	5	2	20	120
French Toast	1 Sl	4	4	15	115
French Toast w/Maple Syrup	1 Sl	4	4	23	150
Fruit Cocktail (Canned)	1 Cup	1	T	47	190
Fruit Cocktail (Fresh)	1 Cup	T	T	35	135
Fruit Drop Candies	3	T	T	10	40
Fruit Punch	6 Ozs	T	T	33	135
Fruit Syrups	1 Tbsp	T	T	14	60
Fudge	1 Oz	T	3	23	120
Fudge, Almond	1 Sq	1	4	22	130
Fudge, Brown Sugar	1 Sq	T	3	22	115
Fudge Cake	1 Serv	6	10	35	255
Fudge, Choc. Candies	1 Pc	T	3	23	120
Fudge Frosting	1 Tbsp	T	3	6	50

	AMT	PRO	FAT	CARB	CALS
Fudge Pop Ice Cream	1	3	6	13	120
Fudge Sauce	1 Tbsp	T	T	18	75
Fudge Sundae Hot	1	7	25	53	465
Garbanzoes (Chick Peas)	4 Ozs	23	5	60	390
Garlic Clove	1	1	T	T	5
Garlic Sauce w/Butter	2 Tbsp	T	33	1	200
Gelatin	2 Ozs	47	T	0	185
Germ, Wheat	1 Oz	7	3	12	100
Gin	2 Ozs	0	0	0	150
Gin Collins	1 Serv	0	0	14	225
Gin Fizz	6 Ozs	0	0	4	125
Gin Rickey	1 Serv	0	0	3	200
Gin & Tonic	6 Ozs	0	0	11	210
Ginger Ale	6 Ozs	0	0	16	75
Ginger Root Fresh	4 Ozs	2	1	8	50
Ginger Snaps	5	1	10	6	165
Gingerbread	1 Sl	2	6	21	180
Goose, Roasted	2 Ozs	13	20	0	240
Goulash, Hungarian	4 Ozs	24	31	4	360
Grape Juice	1/2 Cup	T	T	18	75
Grape Soda	6 Ozs	T	T	28	110
Grapefruit	1/2 Sm	1	T	11	50
Grapefruit, Canned	1/2 Cup	T	T	18	75
Grapefruit, Canned, Swtnd	1/2 Cup	T	T	22	90
Grapefruit Juice, Canned, Unsw	1/2 Cup	T	T	32	65
Grapes	1 Cup	2	2	16	90
Gravy, Chicken	1 Tbsp	T	4	2	50
Green Beans, Canned	4 Ozs	2	T	6	30
Green Beans, Fresh Cooked	1 Cup	2	T	6	30
Green Beans, Frozen	1/2 Cup	2	T	8	40
Green Beans, Raw	1/2 Cup	2	T	8	40
Griddle Cakes	1 Av	2	3	11	80
Grits, Corn	4 Ozs	1	T	12	55
Grits, Hominy	1/2 Cup	2	T	28	120
Gum	1 Stick	0	0	2	8
Gum, Candy Coated	1 Stick	0	0	3	12
Ham	2 Ozs	9	13	0	150
Ham, Baked	2 Ozs	12	12	0	160
Ham, Boiled	2 Oz	10	12	0	150
Ham, Canned Boneless	2 Ozs	10	7	0	107
Ham, Deviled	1 Tbsp	10	10	T	130
Ham Steak	1 Serv	15	5	0	115
Ham, Virginia, Baked	2 Ozs	11	12	0	157
Hamburger, All Beef	2 Ozs	13	11	0	160
Hamburger Rolls	1	3	2	21	120
Hamburger Steak	2 Ozs	13	17	0	276

	AMT	PRO	FAT	CARB	CALS
Hash, Corned Beef	2 Ozs	8	3	4	80
Herbs	1 Tsp	0	0	0	0
Hollandaise Sauce	1 Tbsp	T	8	T	70
Honey	1 Tbsp	T	0	17	65
Horseradish	1 Tsp	T	T	1	5
Hot Dog (No Roll)	1	7	14	0	170
Hot Dog Roll	1	7	6	12	160
Ice Box Cake	1 Sl	3	4	26	165
Ice Box Cookies	3 Med	1	5	19	125
Ice Cream	1/2 Cup	3	9	14	150
Ice Cream,Choc. Cov. Pop	1	3	9	15	150
Ice Cream, Coconut Cov. Pop	1	3	9	18	165
Ice Cream Cone (Cone Alone)	1	2	3	19	110
Ice Cream Fudge Pop	1	3	6	13	120
Ice Cream, Ices	1 Scp	T	T	27	120
Ice Cream Parfait	1	6	15	20	300
Ice Cream Sodas	8 Ozs	3	9	71	285
Ice Cream Sundae	1 Av	7	25	50	450
Ice Cream Sundae (Banana Split)	1 Av	8	25	75	560
Ice Cream Sundae (Hot Fudge)	1 Av	7	25	53	465
Ice, Lemon, Lime, etc.	1 Scp	T	T	27	120
Ice Pop	1	T	T	24	100
Iced Tea (No Sugar or Cream)	1 Gl	T	T	T	2
Icing	1 Tbsp	T	1	11	55
Italian Bread	1 Sl	2	T	12	60
Jams (Most)	1 Tbsp	T	T	14	55
Jellies (Most)	1 Tbsp	T	T	13	55
Jello	1 Serv.	2	0	17	75
Kale	1 Cup	5	0	6	43
Kidney Beans, Cooked	1 Cup	14	T	37	225
Kidney Beans, Raw	1 Cup	26	2	67	380
Kumquats, Candied	1 Oz	T	T	6	25
Kumquats, Fresh	4 Ozs	1	T	17	75
Lamb, Leg of (Roasted)	2 Ozs	15	10	0	160
Lamb Liver	2 Ozs	18	7	1	140
Lamb, Loin Chops of	2 Ozs	13	15	0	192
Lamb Roast	2 Ozs	12	16	0	195
Lamb Shish Kebab	1 Serv	5	4	6	67
Lamb Stew	1 Serv	7	6	7	118
Lard	1 Tbsp	0	12	0	125
Layer Cake	1 Sl	4	5	55	185
Layer, Round w/Icing	1 Sl	6	15	61	400
Leeks	1 Pc	1	T	1	7
Lemon	1	T	T	5	20
Lemon Chiffon Pie	1 Pc	8	14	35	350
Lemon Drops	1 Oz	0	T	28	110

	AMT	PRO	FAT	CARB	CALS
Lemon Frosting	1 Tbsp	T	1	11	55
Lemon Juice	1 Tbsp	T	T	1	5
Lemon Juice (Canned) Swtnd	1/2 Cup	T	T	10	40
Lemon Juice (Canned) Unswtnd	1/2 Cup	T	T	7	30
Lemon Meringue Pie	1 Pc	4	12	45	300
Lemon Peel, Candied	1 Oz	T	T	24	90
Lemon Pudding	1 Serv	3	3	26	140
Lemon Sauce	1 Tbsp	T	1	5	25
Lemon Soda	6 Ozs	0	0	19	80
Lemon Sponge Cake	1 Pc	3	6	54	280
Lemonade	1 Cup	T	T	25	100
Lentil Soup	1 Serv	4	2	40	180
Lentils	1/2 Cup	9	T	17	105
Lettuce	2 Lg Leaves	T	T	1	7
Lettuce Hearts	1/2 Cup	1	T	3	15
Lettuce, Romaine	1/2 Cup	2	T	4	25
Lettuce Shredded	1 Cup	T	T	2	15
Lettuce & Tomato Salad	1 Serv	2	T	6	30
Lichee Nuts, Dried	1 Oz	1	T	15	65
Life Savers (All Flavors)	1 Roll	0	T	30	120
Lima Beans, Canned	4 Ozs	4	T	15	80
Lima Beans (Fresh)	4 Ozs	8	T	27	135
Lime	1	T	T	5	20
Lime Juice, Fresh	1 Cup	0	T	18	60
Lime Juice, Frozen Diluted	4 Ozs	T	T	11	45
Lime Soda	6 Ozs	0	0	19	80
Liver Beef Fried	2 Ozs	15	6	3	130
Liver, Calves, Fried	2 Ozs	15	7	2	140
Liver, Chicken	2 Ozs	15	2	1	92
Liverwurst	2 Ozs	8	15	2	170
Lobster, Baked or Broiled	1 Av	35	11	1	245
Lobster (Canned)	2 Ozs	10	1	T	52
Lobster Newberg	1 Serv	19	11	3	195
Lobster Salad	1/2 Cup	11	7	5	125
Lobster, Steamed	1/2 Av	19	2	T	95
Lobster, Steamed w/2 Tbsp Butter	1 Av	38	26	1	390
Lobster Tails	2 Oz	10	1	T	50
Loganberries (Canned)	1/2 Cup	T	T	20	80
Loganberries, Fresh	1/2 Cup	T	T	11	45
Lollipops	1 Med	0	0	28	115
London Broil	2 Oz	17	4	0	105
Lox	1 Oz	5	5	0	60
Macadamia Nuts	2 Ozs	4	40	9	390
Macaroni Au Gratin	1 Serv	10	12	30	250
Macaroni & Cheese	1 Cup	18	24	43	465
Macaroni,Cooked	4 Ozs	4	T	39	125

	AMT	PRO	FAT	CARB	CALS
Macaroni Salad	1 Cup	4	20	26	260
Mace	1/8 Tsp	0	0	0	0
Malt, Cocoa	1 Cup	10	14	22	255
Mangos, Raw	4 Ozs	T	T	19	75
Manhattan Cocktail	1 Gl	T	T	3	190
Marble Cake	1 Pc	3	5	30	185
Margarine	1 Tbsp	T	11	0	100
Marmalade	1 Tbsp	T	T	14	55
Marshmallow Candy	1 Oz	1	1	23	100
Marshmallow Sauce	1 Tbsp	T	0	6	25
Marshmallow Topping	1 Tbsps	T	0	12	50
Marshmallows	1 Av	T	0	6	25
Martini	3 Ozs	0	0	T	165
Martini, Dry	3 Ozs	0	0	0	205
Matai, Fresh	4 Ozs	2	T	21	90
Mayonnaise	1 Tbsp	T	10	T	90
Meat Balls	2 Ozs	9	8	2	115
Meat Balls & Spaghetti	2 Ozs	4	2	22	75
Meat Gravy	1 Tbsp	T	3	5	50
Meat Loaf	2 Ozs	8	7	1	112
Melba Toast	1 Sl	1	T	4	30
Melon Balls, Frozen	1 Cup	1	T	12	55
Melon, Cantaloupe	1/2	1	T	8	35
Melon, Honeydew	Wedge	T	0	13	50
Milk	1 Cup	9	10	8	170
Milk, Acidophilus	3/4 Cup	8	9	6	145
Milk, Buttermilk	1 Cup	9	T	12	85
Milk, Choc. Flavored	1 Cup	8	8	25	200
Milk, Coconut	1 Cup	4	27	10	300
Milk Condensed, Undiluted	1 Oz	3	3	21	125
Milk, Dry, Nonfat	1 Tbsp	3	T	2	30
Milk, Dry, Whole	1 Tbsp	2	2	3	40
Milk, Goat	1/2 Cup	4	5	5	90
Milk, Skimmed	1 Cup	9	T	13	85
Milk, Skimmed, Choc.	1 Cup	8	T	26	130
Milk, Soy Bean	1 Cup	8	3	5	80
Milk, Whole	1 Cup	9	10	12	175
Mince Pie	1 Sl	3	9	52	300
Minestrone	1 Cup	4	3	10	80
Mint, Chopped	1 Tbsp	0	0	0	0
Mint Leaves	1 Tbsp	0	0	0	0
Mixed Vegetables (Canned)	4 Ozs	4	T	15	75
Mixed Vegetables (Frozen)	4 Ozs	4	T	16	75
Molasses, Blackstrap	1 Tbsp	T	T	11	45
Molasses, Cane Syrup	1 Tbsp	T	T	13	50
Molasses, Cookie	1	T	1	5	35

	AMT	PRO	FAT	CARB	CALS
Mousse	1 Serv	4	30	17	355
Muffins	1 Av	4	5	19	135
Muffins, Blueberry	1 Av	4	5	23	150
Muffins, Bran	1 Av	4	5	24	150
Muffins, Cinnamon	1 Av	2	4	23	135
Muffins, Date	1 Av	4	5	41	140
Muffins, English	1 Av	4	5	21	150
Muffins, Raisin	1 Av	4	4	27	160
Muffins, White	1 Av	3	2	21	120
Muffins, Whole Wheat	1 Av	2	3	19	115
Mushroom Soup, Creamed	1 Cup	2	13	13	180
Mushrooms	1/2 Cup	3	T	5	35
Mushrooms, Broild w/Tsp. But	1/2 Cup	2	5	3	65
Mushrooms, Button	1/2 Cup	2	T	3	20
Mushrooms, Canned	1/2 Cup	2	T	3	20
Mushrooms, Cooked Fresh	1/2 Cup	2	1	3	30
Mushrooms, Creamed	1/2 Cup	3	2	3	42
Muskmelon	Av Serv	1	T	8	30
Mussels	2 Ozs	5	1	0	37
Mustard	1 Tbsp	T	T	T	10
Mustard, Dry	1 Tbsp	T	T	T	10
Mustard Greens	1 Cup	3	T	5	30
Mustard, Prepared	1 Tbsp	T	T	T	10
Mustard Sauce	1/4 Cup	2	6	6	85
Mutton, Boiled	2 Ozs	13	15	0	187
Mutton Chop	2 Ozs	13	15	0	187
Mutton Chops or Roast	2 Ozs	12	16	0	195
Mutton, Leg Roast	2 Ozs	10	14	0	162
Napoleons	1 Av	7	15	30	300
Nectarine	1	1	T	12	50
Noodles, Butter Cheese	1 Serv	9	13	10	195
Nut Bread, Date	1 Sl	2	1	21	100
Nut Brittle	2 Ozs	4	6	45	250
Nutmeg	1/8 Tsp	0	0	0	0
Nuts, Brazil, Shelled	2 Ozs	8	35	6	365
Nuts, Butter	5 Av	2	4	1	50
Nuts, Cashew	7 Av	2	6	4	75
Nuts, Hazel	2 Ozs	8	37	9	380
Nuts, Hickory	10 Av	2	9	2	100
Nuts, Macadamia	2 Ozs	4	40	9	390
Nuts, Peanuts	10	6	11	3	175
Nuts, Pine	2 Ozs	17	27	7	310
Nuts, Pistachio	16	2	5	2	50
Oat Cereal, Ready to Eat	1/2 Cup	4	1	13	75
Oatmeal, Cooked	1 Cup	5	3	25	150
Oatmeal Cookies	1 Lg	2	3	15	90

	AMT	PRO	FAT	CARB	CALS
Oil, Salad	1 Tbsp	T	14	0	125
Oil, Unsaturated, Vegetable	1 Tbsp	0	14	0	125
Oil & Vinegar Dressing	1 Tbsp	T	14	0	125
Okra	1 Cup	3	T	10	50
Okra, Cooked	8 Pods	2	T	6	30
Olive Oil	1 Tbsp	T	14	0	125
Olives, Green	2 Ozs	T	7	1	65
Olives, Ripe	2 Ozs	T	8	1	75
Omelet	2 Eggs	11	12	T	150
Omelet, Asparagus	2 Eggs	16	14	6	220
Omelet, Cheese	2 Egg	18	21	1	260
Omelet, Jelly	2 Eggs	12	34	13	405
Omelet, Mushroom	2 Eggs	12	12	2	160
Omelet, Onion	2 Eggs	11	12	1	160
Omelet, Plain	2 Eggs	11	12	1	155
Omelet, Spanish	2 Eggs	12	13	8	200
Onion Roll	1	3	2	23	130
Onion Soup (Clear)	1 Cup	5	1	4	50
Onion Soup, French	4 Ozs	5	2	5	60
Onions, Boiled	1 Cup	1	T	7	30
Onions, Creamed	1/2 Cup	3	4	8	65
Onions, French Fried	1 Lg	2	15	10	175
Onions, Fried	1 Lg	2	15	10	175
Onions, Green	6 Sm	T	T	T	25
Onions, Raw	1	2	T	11	50
Onions, Raw (Bermuda)	4 Ozs	2	T	10	40
Onions, Raw Chopped	1	2	T	11	50
Orange	1 Med	1	T	17	70
Orange Juice (Canned) Swtnd	1 Cup	2	T	31	140
Orange Juice (Canned) Unswtnd	1 Cup	1	T	26	110
Orange Juice, Florida	1 Cup	2	T	26	110
Orange Mandarin	1 Med	1	T	10	50
Orange Marmalade	1 Tbsp	T	T	14	55
Orange Peel, Candied	2 Ozs	T	T	48	190
Orange Sections	1/2 Cup	1	T	11	50
Orange-Grapefruit Juice	1 Cup	3	2	20	110
Orangeade Juice	1/2 Cup	1	T	19	80
Oregano	1/8 Tsp	0	0	0	0
Oyster, Blue Point	12	12	2	7	100
Oyster, Cape Cod	6	12	2	5	100
Oyster Cocktail, Raw	6 Med	9	1	6	75
Oyster Crackers	1/2 Oz	1	2	10	60
Oyster, Fried	2 Ozs	5	8	10	135
Oyster Stew w/Milk	1 Cup	5	5	21	150
Oysters on the Half Shell	6 Med	10	2	6	75
Oysters, Scalloped	6	12	8	6	150

	AMT	PRO	FAT	CARB	CALS
Pancakes, Blueberry	2	8	8	29	250
Pancakes, Buckwheat	1	6	8	21	175
Pancakes, Choc.	2	2	8	16	200
Pancakes, Griddle	1	2	3	11	80
Pancakes, Wheat	1	2	3	11	80
Pancakes, Wheat (Enriched Flour)	1	2	3	11	80
Papaya	4 Ozs	T	T	11	45
Papaya Marmalade	1 Tbsp	T	T	15	55
Parfaits	1 Av	6	15	14	215
Parsley	1 Tbsp	T	T	T	1
Parsnips, Cooked	1 Cup	2	1	21	95
Passion Fruit	4 Ozs	2	1	35	155
Pastry, Danish	1 Pc	4	13	25	240
Pate de Fois Gras	1 Tbsp	2	8	1	85
Pate Maison	1 Oz	3	13	T	130
Pea Beans, Dried, Cooked	4 Ozs	4	T	18	90
Pea Soup	1 Cup	3	1	16	85
Peach Brandy	Shot	T	T	7	100
Peach Pie	Av Serv	3	11	70	390
Peach Short Cake	Av Serv	6	12	41	300
Peaches (Canned)	2 Hlvs	T	T	11	45
Peaches (Canned in Water)	2 Hlvs	T	T	9	35
Peaches, Dried	2 Hlvs	4	T	76	300
Peaches, Fresh	1 Med	1	T	11	50
Peanut Bar Candy	2 Ozs	5	8	17	160
Peanut Brittle	2 Ozs	3	6	46	140
Peanut Butter Spread	1 Tbsp	4	8	3	100
Peanut Cookie	1	1	2	9	65
Peanuts	10	6	11	3	175
Pear	1 Av	1	T	18	75
Pear Juice Nectar	4 Ozs	T	T	12	50
Pears, Canned	2 Hlvs	T	T	17	70
Pears, Canned (Water-packed)	2 Hlvs	T	T	9	35
Peas, Black-Eyed, Canned, Drained	4 Ozs	8	1	17	110
Peas, Canned	1 Cup	5	T	19	100
Peas, Chick (Garbanzos Dry)	1/2 Cup	23	5	60	390
Peas, Fresh	Av Serv	3	T	10	55
Peas, Green	Av Serv	4	T	14	75
Pecan Pie	1 Av Sl	6	25	58	470
Pecans	6	1	7	2	75
Pecans, Chopped	1 Tbsp	T	3	1	35
Pecans (Halves)	2 Ozs	5	40	8	290
Pepper	1/8 Tsp	0	0	0	0
Pepper, Cayenne	1/8 Tsp	0	0	0	0
Peppermint Candy, Choc. Covered	1 Oz	T	3	21	115
Peppermint Patties	1 Oz	T	1	25	105

	AMT	PRO	FAT	CARB	CALS
Peppers, Fresh	1 Med	1	T	4	20
Peppers, Stuffed	1	14	6	11	155
Perch	2 Ozs	11	2	0	60
Perch, Sea	2 Ozs	11	0	0	50
Persimmons	1 Av	1	T	24	100
Pheasant, Roasted	1 Serv	24	5	0	150
Pickles, Dill or Sour	1 Lg	T	T	3	10
Pickles, Sweet	1 Sm	T	T	5	20
Pie, See By Name	Av Pc	T	6	75	350
Pig Brains	Av Serv	6	5	1	70
Pig Liver	Av Serv	11	2	1	65
Pig's Feet, Pickled	2 Ozs	9	8	T	112
Pike	Av Serv	21	1	0	95
Pimiento, Hot	1/2 Cup	1	T	6	30
Pimientoes	1/2 Cup	1	T	6	30
Pina Colada	1	6	0	31	245
Pineapple, Candied	1 Sl	T	T	30	120
Pineapple, Canned	1 Sl	T	T	12	50
Pineapple, Canned, Low Calorie	1/2 Cup	T	T	11	45
Pineapple, Crushed (Canned)	1/2 Cup	5	8	15	150
Pineapple, Fresh	1 Cup	T	T	16	60
Pineapple Upside Down Cake	1 Pc	7	10	38	275
Pinto Beans	1/2 Cup	25	1	72	390
Pita, shell	1	4	1	13	70
Pizza Pie w/Cheese	1 Pc	14	9	25	240
Pizza, Sausage	1 Pc	9	10	23	265
Plums, Fresh	1	1	T	7	30
Popcorn, Air popped	1 Cup	1	T	10	50
Popcorn, No Butter	1 Cup	2	1	11	55
Popcorn, Sugar Coated	1 Cup	1	T	11	55
Popcorn w/1 Tbsp. Butter	1 Cup	2	12	11	155
Popovers	Av	3	3	11	75
Poppy Seeds	1/8 Tsp	0	0	0	0
Pork Chops	1 Med	30	16	0	275
Pork Chops, Fried	1 Med	30	41	0	375
Pork Chops, Loin Ctr Cut, Broiled	1 Med	30	16	0	275
Pork Cured, Bacon	2 Ozs	4	38	T	375
Pork Cured Ham	2 Ozs	10	6	0	107
Pork, Heart	2 Ozs	9	2	T	65
Pork, Kidney	1 Serv	9	2	1	57
Pork, Leg Roast	2 Ozs	7	19	0	225
Pork Liver	Av Serv	11	2	2	75
Pork, Loin (Roasted)	Av Serv	13	16	0	202
Pork, Spiced	2 Ozs	8	14	0	157
Pot Roast	4 Ozs	32	17	0	290
Potato Au Gratin	4 Ozs	6	9	16	165

	AMT	PRO	FAT	CARB	CALS
Potato, Baked	4 Ozs	4	T	28	125
Potato, Boiled	4 Ozs	4	T	28	125
Potato Chips	1/2 Cup	1	8	7	100
Potato, French Fried	6 Av	1	5	12	100
Potato, Idaho Baked	1 Med	4	T	28	125
Potato, Irish, Boiled	1 Med	4	T	28	125
Potato Julienne	1 Med	8	6	30	225
Potato, Mashed	1/2 Cup	2	3	16	90
Potato Pan Browned	4 Ozs	2	13	33	260
Potato Salad	4 Ozs	3	11	16	175
Potato Soup, Cream of	4 Ozs	4	5	8	100
Potato, Sweet, Baked	5 Ozs	3	1	45	200
Potato, Sweet, Boiled	5 Ozs	2	1	44	160
Potato, Sweet, Candied	6 Ozs	2	5	60	295
Potatoes, Fried	1/2 Cup	4	16	12	285
Potatoes, Hashed Brown	4 Ozs	3	13	33	260
Potatoes, Scalloped	1/2 Cup	3	4	14	120
Potatoes, Sweet, Canned	1 Cup	5	1	45	285
Pound Cake	1 Sl	3	6	35	380
Prune Juice	4 Ozs	1	T	23	94
Prunes, Cooked (Sugar Added)	4 Ozs	1	T	50	205
Prunes, Dried	4	1	T	24	100
Prunes, Stewed (No Sugar)	4 Ozs	1	T	40	165
Pudding, Bread	1/2 Cup	6	7	32	210
Pudding, Butterscotch	1/2 Cup	3	3	23	140
Pudding, Cornstarch	1/2 Cup	3	3	24	135
Pudding, Date	1/2 Cup	4	5	16	125
Pumpkin (Canned)	1 Cup	2	1	18	90
Pumpkin Pie	1 Pc	8	23	47	430
Pumpkin Seeds	1 Oz	8	13	4	155
Quail, Broiled	2 Ozs	14	4	0	95
Quince, Fresh	1	T	T	12	50
Quinine Water	6 Ozs	0	0	12	50
Rabbit	2 Ozs	34	11	0	120
Rabbit Stew	2 Ozs	7	6	7	117
Radishes	4 Sm	T	T	2	8
Raisin Bran Flakes	1 Cup	4	T	40	140
Raisin Bread	1 Sl	2	1	12	65
Raisin Cookies	1/4 lb.	5	6	90	430
Raisins	1/4 Cup	1	T	29	120
Raspberries	1 Cup	2	2	16	80
Raspberry Pie	Av Sl	T	6	57	280
Relish, Pickle, Sweet	1 Tbsp	T	T	3	12
Rhubarb	1 Cup Diced	1	T	5	18
Rhubarb,Frozen	1/2 Cup	1	T	20	80
Rice, Boiled White	1 Cup	4	T	49	223

	AMT	PRO	FAT	CARB	CALS
Rice, Brown	1 Cup	3	T	38	178
Rice,Spanish	1 Cup	4	4	40	210
Rice, Wild, Cooked	1 Cup	6	2	30	70
Roast Beef	2 Ozs	16	5	0	114
Roast Beef (Canned)	2 Ozs	14	6	0	125
Roast Beef Hash	2 Ozs	5	6	6	102
Roll, Plain	1	3	2	21	120
Root Beer	6 Ozs	0	0	15	75
Rosemary	1/8 Tsp	0	0	0	0
Rum	1 Shot	T	T	T	100
Rutabaga	1/2 Cup	1	T	9	40
Ry-Krisp	3	2	T	10	50
Rye Bread	1 Sl	2	T	12	55
Rye Flour, Dark	1 Cup	20	3	76	410
Rye Flour, Light	1 Cup	11	1	98	440
Rye Wafer Crackers	1	T	T	2	8
Sage	1/8 Tsp	0	0	0	0
Salami	2 Ozs	14	22	T	240
Sauerkraut	1/2 Cup	1	T	5	25
Sausage (Canned) Pork	2 Ozs	10	18	1	212
Sausage, Frankfurter, Cooked	1	6	15	1	165
Sausage, Knockwurst	1 Av	12	16	1	185
Sausage, Liverwurst	1 Sl	5	7	T	90
Sausage, Polish	2 Ozs	9	14	0	170
Sausage, Pork	1	10	25	0	265
Sausage, Pork Dried	2 Ozs	18	21	0	242
Sausage, Vienna Canned	2 Oz	8	11	0	135
Scallions	5	1	T	5	20
Scallops	2 Ozs	14	1	1	70
Scallops, Broiled	2 Ozs	14	1	1	70
Scallops, Fried w/Batter	3-4	20	9	15	230
Scotch	Shot	0	0	0	100
Scotch & Soda	1 Drink	0	0	0	100
Seltzer (Carbonated Water)	4 Ozs	0	0	0	0
Seltzer Water	8 Ozs	0	0	0	0
Sesame Seeds, Whole	1 Oz	5	14	6	165
Shad, Roe	2 Ozs	12	1	0	65
Sherbet Ice Cream, w/Water	1/4 Pt	1	1	35	130
Shoofly Pie	1 Pc	5	8	48	285
Short Bread	1 Sl	2	7	19	140
Short Cake, Banana	1 Sl	4	7	44	250
Short Cake, Biscuit	1	4	10	27	210
Short Cake, Peach	Av Serv	6	12	41	300
Short Cake, Plain	Av Serv	5	11	31	255
Short Cake, Raspberry	Av Serv	69	12	47	325
Short Cake, Strawberry	Av Serv	6	12	43	300

	AMT	PRO	FAT	CARB	CALS
Shortening, Crisco	1 Tbsp	0	14	0	125
Shrimp, Boiled	2 Ozs	10	0	1	45
Shrimp, Canned	2 Ozs	14	0	T	66
Shrimp Cocktail	6 Med Size	16	1	1	75
Shrimp Creole	2 Ozs	10	4	2	92
Shrimp, French Fried	10 Av	23	12	11	240
Shrimp, Fried	3 Jumbo	8	4	8	100
Shrimp Salad Sandwich	1	14	2	26	180
Shrimp Salad w/Celery	1 Serv	10	1	5	70
Shrimp Scampi in Garlic Butter	6	20	24	T	300
Snails	6 Med	16	13	2	190
Soda, Cherry	6 Ozs	0	0	21	80
Soda,Chocolate	6 Ozs	0	0	15	75
Soda Crackers	6	5	6	35	215
Soda, Cream	6 Ozs	0	0	21	75
Soda, Ginger Ale	6 Ozs	0	0	16	75
Soda, Grape	6 Ozs	0	0	28	110
Soda, Ice Cream	10 Ozs	3	9	71	285
Soda, Lemon	6 Ozs	0	0	19	80
Soda, Lime	6 Ozs	0	0	19	80
Soda, Orange	6 Oz	0	0	19	80
Sorghum Syrup	3 Ozs	T	T	58	230
Souffle, Almond	1/2 Cup	17	6	40	280
Souffle, Cheese	1/2 Cup	11	19	6	240
Sour Balls	6	0	T	28	110
Sour Cream	1 Tbsp	T	3	T	30
Soy Beans	1/2 Cup	11	6	6	120
Soy Sauce	1 Tsp	T	T	1	4
Soybean Curd	1 Oz	2	1	3	20
Soybean Milk	8 Ozs	8	3	5	80
Soybean Sprouts, Raw	1/2 Cup	7	2	3	70
Soybeans, Mature-Dried	1/2 Cup	25	T	25	180
Spaghetti, Cooked	1 Cup	7	1	46	200
Spaghetti w/2 Meatballs	4 Ozs	8	5	45	150
Spaghetti w/Butter	4 Ozs	4	9	20	210
Spaghetti w/Clam Sauce	4 Ozs	8	1	43	220
Spaghetti w/Meat Sauce	4 Ozs	5	3	47	235
Spaghetti w/Tomato Sauce	4 Ozs	3	1	47	210
Spareribs, Barbecues	6 Av	24	47	0	505
Spareribs, Pork	2 Ozs	11	22	0	247
Spinach	1/2 Cup	3	T	3	25
Spinach (Canned)	1 Cup	6	1	6	55
Spinach , Frozen	1 Cup	7	1	6	60
Spinach, Raw	1 Cup	7	1	6	60
Spinach Souffle	Av Serv	9	12	6	170
Sponge Cake	Av Pc	2	2	22	115

	AMT	PRO	FAT	CARB	CALS
Squab	1	20	8	0	160
Squash, Acorn	1/2 Cup	T	T	12	50
Squash,Butternut	1/2 Cup	1	T	12	55
Squash, Hubbard	1/2 Cup	1	T	10	50
Squash, Summer	1/2 Cup	1	T	4	20
Squash, Winter, Boiled	1/2 Cup	1	T	10	45
Squid	2 Ozs	9	0	1	45
Steak, Chopped	1/4 Lb	31	13	0	245
Steak, Chuck w/Bone	2 Ozs	20	5	0	125
Steak, Cube	2 Ozs	12	23	0	260
Steak, Flank	2 Ozs	11	6	0	100
Steak, Ham	2 Ozs	16	5	0	115
Steak, Pepper	2 Ozs	15	6	2	125
Steak, Porterhouse	2 Ozs	11	23	0	260
Steak, Rib	2 Ozs	16	9	0	142
Steak, Round	2 Ozs	11	6	0	100
Steak,Salisbury	2 Ozs	19	11	T	122
Steak,Sirloin	2 Ozs	18	4	0	112
Steak,Swiss	2 Ozs	17	4	7	105
Steak,T-Bone	2 Ozs	11	24	0	260
Steak, Tenderloin	2 Ozs	17	6	0	120
Steak,Veal	2 Ozs	20	7	0	132
Stew, Beef	2 Ozs	3	2	3	50
Stew, Beef & Vegetable	2 Ozs	3	2	3	50
Stew, Irish	2 Ozs	7	6	7	117
Strawberries	1 Cup	1	1	12	55
String Beans	1/2 Cup	2	T	6	30
Strogonoff, Beef	2 Ozs	19	10	3	182
Stuffed Cabbage	Av Serv	15	6	7	140
Stuffed Peppers	1	14	6	11	155
Stuffing,Bread	1/2 Cup	5	14	28	280
Stuffing, Chestnut	1/2 Cup	4	7	26	185
Succotash	1/2 Cup	5	T	21	110
Sugar, Beet	1 Tsp	0	0	4	18
Sugar, Brown	1 Tsp	0	0	4	18
Sugar, Cane	1 Tsp	0	0	4	18
Sugar Cookie	1	1	2	7	50
Sugar, Granulated	1 Tsp	0	0	4	50
Sugar, Maple	1 Oz	0	0	12	100
Sugar, Powdered	1 Tbsp	0	0	24	90
Sunflower Seeds	1 Oz	7	14	6	159
Syrup,Brown Sugar	1 Tbsp	0	0	15	60
Syrup, Caramel	1 Tbsp	0	0	16	65
Syrup, Choc	1 Tbsp	T	T	10	35
Syrup, Corn	1 Tbsp	T	T	12	50
Syrup, Maple	1 Tbsp	0	0	13	50

	AMT	PRO	FAT	CARB	CALS
Syrup, Molasses	1 Tbsp	T	T	11	55
Tangerine	1 Lg	1	T	8	35
Tangerine Juice, Fresh	1/2 Cup	1	T	10	50
Tapioca, Pudding	1/2 Cup	6	6	24	175
Tapioca, Ready-to-Serve	1/2 Cup	5	5	19	150
Tarragon	1/8 Tsp	0	0	0	0
Tartar Sauce	1 Tbsp	T	8	T	75
Tarts, Apple	1	2	7	26	175
Tarts, Blueberry	1	2	7	21	150
Tea	1 Cup	T	T	T	2
Tea, Iced, No Sugar or Cream	1 Gl	T	T	T	2
Thyme	1/8 Tsp	0	0	0	0
Toast, French,1 Tbsp. Maple Syrup	1 Pc	4	4	23	150
Toddy, Hot	1 Cup	2	3	24	150
Tofu	4 Oz	10	6	1	90
Toll House Cookie	3 Med	2	6	22	150
Tomato Consomme	1 Serv	3	3	6	65
Tomato, Fresh	Med	1	T	4	20
Tomato Juice	1 Cup	2	T	10	50
Tomato & Lettuce Salad	1 Serv	2	T	6	30
Tomato Soup, Clear	1 Serv	T	T	4	15
Tomato Soup, Creamed	1 Serv	6	6	18	155
Tomatoes, Stewed or Canned	1 Cup	3	T	10	50
Tortilla	1	1	1	10	55
Tortoni, Biscuit	1 Sm	2	12	14	175
Tuna	2 Ozs	12	8	0	85
Tuna, Canned in Oil, Drained	2 Ozs	11	3	0	79
Tuna, Canned in Water	2 Ozs	14	T	0	63
Tuna Salad	1/2 Cup	16	12	2	180
Turkey	2 Ozs	18	5	0	125
Turkey, All Dark	2 Ozs	16	4	0	115
Turkey, All White	2 Ozs	18	2	0	100
Turkey (Canned, Boned)	2 Ozs	12	7	0	112
Turkey, Cream of, Soup	1 Cup	16	10	12	200
Turkey Hash	2 Ozs	7	6	4	72
Turkey, Roasted	2 Ozs	18	5	0	125
Turkey Soup	1 Cup	2	1	13	70
Turnip Greens (Canned)	1 Cup	3	1	11	55
Turnip Greens, Cooked	1 Cup	4	T	8	45
Turnips, Cooked	1 Cup	2	T	12	55
V-8 Juice	1Cup	2	T	9	45
Vanilla Extract	1 Tsp	1	T	0	5
Vanilla Ice Cream	1 Scp	3	9	14	150
Vanilla Malted w/Ice Cream	1 Cup	10	10	53	235
Vanilla Soda w/Ice Cream	8 Ozs	3	9	71	285
Vanilla Wafer Cookie	1 Av	T	1	4	25

	AMT	PRO	FAT	CARB	CALS
Veal Chop	1 Med	30	15	0	260
Veal Cutlet, Breaded	2 Ozs	12	5	4	115
Veal Cutlet, Broiled	2 Ozs	16	6	0	116
Veal Loaf	2 Ozs	10	6	1	117
Veal & Peppers	2 Ozs	8	6	0	90
Veal Roast	2 Ozs	15	9	0	122
Veal Steak	2 Ozs	20	7	0	132
Vermicelli	1/2 Cup	3	4	8	80
Vermouth	2 Ozs	0	0	3	60
Vichyssoise	1 Cup	6	20	15	275
Vienna Bread	1 Sl	2	1	10	60
Vinegar	1 Oz	T	T	1	5
Vodka	1 Oz	0	0	T	70
Waffle, Blueberry	1 Med	9	10	35	300
Waffle, Choc	1 Med	11	17	48	380
Waffle, Ham	1 Med	18	20	28	325
Waffle, Plain	1 Med	10	12	28	225
Walnuts	10	11	28	8	355
Water	1 Cup	0	0	0	0
Watercress	1 Bunch	2	T	3	20
Watermelon	Med Sl	1	T	22	100
Welsh Rabbit	1/2 Cup	18	30	22	430
Wheat, Cream of	1/2 Cup	2	T	15	65
Wheat Flour, All Purpose	1 Cup	13	1	85	400
Wheat, Thin, Cracker	4	1	2	5	55
Whipped Cream	1 Cup	3	45	4	420
Whiskey	1 Shot	T	T	T	100
White Sauce, Med	1 Tbsp	1	2	1	25
Wine, Red	1 Gl	T	0	4	75
Wine, White	1 Gl	T	0	2	75
Worcestershire Sauce	1 Tbsp	T	0	2	10
Yam Canned	8 Ozs	2	T	54	225
Yam Potatoes, Baked	1 Sm	1	T	23	105
Yams, Candied	1 Med	2	5	60	300
Yeast, Bakers, Dry	1 Oz	10	T	3	85
Yeast, Dry, Brewers	1 Tbsp	5	T	3	50
Yogurt-Read All Containers	1 Cup	7	8	13	140
Zucchini	8 Ozs	2	T	8	40
Zwieback	1 Av	T	T	5	30

biographies

Victoria Zak is a writer, lecturer, and marketing consultant specializing in the health care field. She has worked with the country's leading experts on the combined-science approach to weight loss and fitness, developing diet systems, videotapes, and educational materials, including the *Obesity Lose to Win* video and *Rx Weight Control* newsletter. Her articles have appeared in many publications including **Shape, Ladies Home Journal** and **USA Today**. Her most recent book was **The Fat-to-Muscle Diet** by Putnam.

Peter Vash, MD, MPH is an endocrinologist and an internist on the clinical faculty of the University of California Los Angeles Medical Center. He is a trustee and officer of the American Society of Bariatric Physicians, and maintains a private practice in Century City, California, where he specializes in treatment of obesity and eating disorders. His most recent book was **The Fat-to-Muscle Diet** by Putnam.

Deborah D. Reilly is an entrepreneur in the diet and fitness field. She has owned two diet and exercise centers in New Jersey and personally counselled thousands of people in weight loss, maintenance and fitness techniques. Prior to developing her own businesses, she was in casino management in Atlantic City in Trump Plaza. Her education and background was in physical education and nutrition.

"The Dieter's Dictionary is an excellent resource for anyone who is moving from a self-deprived, powerless model of relating to food to a self-nurturing choice model of relating to food."

Margaret H. Perryman, MSW, ACSW
Creator of "*Breaking The Binge-Diet Cycle*" Training